PAEDIATRIC GASTROENTEROLOGY

DR. AHMED IZZELDIN ABUELGASIM

authorHOUSE®

AuthorHouse™ UK
1663 Liberty Drive
Bloomington, IN 47403 USA
www.authorhouse.co.uk
Phone: 0800 047 8203 (Domestic TFN)
+44 1908 723714 (International)

© 2020 DR. AHMED IZZELDIN ABUELGASIM. *All rights reserved.*

No part of this book may be reproduced, stored in a retrieval system, or transmitted by any means without the written permission of the author.

Published by AuthorHouse 03/17/2020

ISBN: 978-1-7283-9986-7 (sc)
ISBN: 978-1-7283-9987-4 (hc)
ISBN: 978-1-7283-9985-0 (e)

Print information available on the last page.

Any people depicted in stock imagery provided by Getty Images are models, and such images are being used for illustrative purposes only.
Certain stock imagery © Getty Images.

This book is printed on acid-free paper.

Because of the dynamic nature of the Internet, any web addresses or links contained in this book may have changed since publication and may no longer be valid. The views expressed in this work are solely those of the author and do not necessarily reflect the views of the publisher, and the publisher hereby disclaims any responsibility for them.

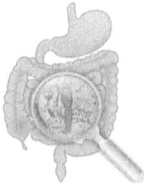

This comprehensive handbook provides an essential source of information and practical advice for medical students, trainee and pediatric residents. Although the development of information via the internet has made it easy to learn , find information and communications, yet this handbook has collected most of the essential information needed about gastrointestinal disorder during childhood.

As in most of my handbook, this book also starts with congenital malformation of the gastrointestinal tract.

Problems that arise from the congenital malformation present very early in infancy as surgical emergency situation that threaten lives if not managed promptly.

An important chapter in this handbook is the Functional Gastro-intestinal disorder of infancy. These are very common problems affecting about half the population of infant across the globe. They comprise a range of recurrent disorders that are explained by anatomical , structural or biochemical abnormalities. Acquired gastrointestinal disorders are mentioned in details so as the inflammatory bowel diseases.

Vomiting is a major symptoms in children of all age groups and so I have chaptered it separately in this handbook.

Diarrhea is one of the most common illness among children in developing countries with 1.5 billion episodes of diarrhea and 4 million associated deaths among children each year. This is why it is important to be familiar with its causes of which foods poisoning is part of and method of treatment.

Malabsoption Syndrome are disorders affecting the digestion and absorption of nutrients key to survival.

Key to dehydration management is prevention of dehydration and promotion of rehydration in those already dehydrated. Failure in management is the major cause of morbidity and mortality in gastro enteritis cases.

Accurate diagnosis of defecation disorders impacts treatment outcomes. This can be achieved through the accurate recording of key information gathered from history, examinations, discussion with patients about family history and dietary habits.

Liver disease developments is silent with no signs or symptoms and one of the leading causes of premature death in England responsible for more than 1 in 10 deaths of people in their 40's.

This book is a summation of the knowledge culminated from 40 + experience in the specialty as a consultant pediatricians and a fundamental reference to people passionate about medicine.

Dr. Ahmed Izzeldin Abuelgassim
Consultant Peadreician
United Arab Emirates

Email Address: ahmed.gassim@hotmail.co.uk

March 2020

CONTENTS

Gastrointestinal Tract 1
Functional Gastro-intestinal Disorders during Infancy........................21
Acquired Gastrointestinal Disorders 35
Inflammatory Bowel Disease...47
Vomiting..53
Diarrhoeal Diseases...57
Malabsorption Syndrome 89
Coeliac Disease..99
Cystic Fibrosis 103
Dehydration 107
Defecation Disorders..115
Acute Abdominal Pain 121
Acute Hepatitis 123
Liver Transplantation 135

ANALYTICAL CONTENTS

Congenital Malformations 1
Cleft Lip and Cleft Palate 1
Pierre Robin Syndrome 2
Tongue Tie 2
Oesophageal Atresia and Tracheo-Oesophageal Fistula.................3
Diaphragmatic Hernia..4
Hiatus Hernia..5
Congenital Hypertrophic Pyloric Stenosis 6
Congenital Duodenal Obstruction...7
Congenital Intestinal Obstruction below the Duodenum 9
Atresia of the Jejunum and Ileum...9
Meconium Ileus..10
Meconium Peritonitis..11
Malrotation of the Gut with or Without Volvulus 11
Meckel's Diverticulum...12
Duplication of the Gastrointestinal Tract......................................13
Hirschsprung Disease..14
Congenital Anorectal Malformation 15
Abdominal Wall Malformations 15
Umbilical Hernia..16
Omphalocele 16
Gastroschisis...17
Inguinal Hernia 17
Intestinal Polyps 18
Familial Polyposis of the Colon..18
Peutz-Jeghers Syndrome 18
Gardner Syndrome...19
Functional Gastro-intestinal Disorders (FGIDs) 22

Infant Regurgitation..22
Functional Constipation...24
Infantile colic..27
Functional diarrhea...30
Dyschezia..31
Rumination syndrome..32
Cyclic Vomiting Syndrome (CVS)..33
Acute Stomatitis..35
Gastroesophageal Reflux Disease..37
Peptic Ulcer...40
Intussusception...41
Acute Appendicitis..43
Peritonitis..44
Achalasia of the Oesophagus..46
Crohn's Disease...48
Ulcerative Colitis...48
Gastrointestinal bleeding..51
Haematemesis...51
Malaenia and passing fresh blood per rectum.........................52
Acute Diarrhoea..62
Viral Gastro enteritis...62
Bacterial Gastroenteritis...65
Parasitic gastro enteritis..71
Antibiotic-associated colitis..75
Food Poisoning...76
Chronic Diarrhoea..81
Disorder of Disaccharide Absorption......................................92
Cow's Milk Protein Intolerance...95
Acrodermatitis Enteropathica..105
Familial Chloride Diarrhoea..105
Constipation...115
Encopresis...118
Fulminant Hepatic Failure...127
Reye's Syndrome...129
Wilson Disease (Hepatolenticular Degeneration)................129
Cirrhosis of the Liver...130
Portal Hypertension...133
Acute Pancreatitis...136

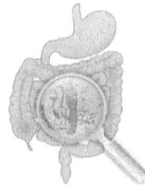

GASTROINTESTINAL TRACT

Gastrointestinal problems are very common in paediatric practice. They could endanger life if not diagnosed and managed early specifically. Detailed history and careful examination will enable doctors to reach a diagnosis. Most problems can be corrected either medically or surgically.

Congenital Malformations

Cleft Lip and Cleft Palate

- Genetic and environmental factors are the underlying aetiology.
- This defect is common with an incidence in some studies of 1:700 live birth.
- Cleft lip and cleft palate may occur singly or together.
- They can be unilateral or bilateral.
- Cleft lip alone is more common in males. Associated malformations that might be seen with cleft lip include hypertelorism, heart, foot and hand malformations.
- The cleft palate can involve just the alveolar ridge or the ridge and entire palate. Clefts can also be isolated soft palate defects. A bifid uvula might indicate a sub mucous cleft.
- Only the most severe degrees of cleft palate interfere with sucking. In such cases, feeding can be by a spoon or a long soft nipple with a large hole, or by using a feeding aid and orthodontic appliance.
- Cleft lip should be repaired during the first three months of life.

- Cleft palate surgical repair is performed between 15-24 months of age. These children are subject to recurrent otitis media, nasopharyngitis, speech problems and teeth problems.
- Speech therapy should be started soon after successful operation to prevent the cleft palate type of speech which has a muffled tone with a normal quality voice.

Pierre Robin Syndrome

This is a triad of micrognathia, glossoptosis and high arched or cleft palate.

- It could be familial or sporadic in occurrence.
- The primary defect is hypoplasia of the mandible which results in backward displacement of the attachments of the genoglossi causing glossoptosis. This allows the tongue to fall backwards and downwards obstructing the oropharynx.
- It results in feeding problems as well as airway obstruction with stridor, cyanotic attacks and inhalation pneumonia.
- Infants have typical "shrew face" with a receding chin.
- The main objective of treatment is to prevent asphyxia until the mandible grows and be able to accommodate the tongue.
- The infant is nursed in the prone position. If this fails an oral airway should be used. In severe cases intubation and tracheotomy maybe needed. Glossopexy has shown some degree of success.
- The cleft palate can be repaired later.
- Associated malformations include Strickler Syndrome, Treacher Collins Syndrome and Velocardiofacial which is a deletion of chromosome 22q11.

Tongue Tie

- The tongue is connected to the floor of the mouth by the lingual frenum. If the attachment is tight and high up on the alveolar ridge, it is called ankyloglossia or tongue tie.
- The short frenulum prevents both protrusion and elevation of the tongue. It does not interfere with speech development.

- In mild cases treatment consists of reassurance.
- Frenulectomy maybe recommended if there is a question of suckling difficulties or dental health when the tongue cannot be used for clearing food from around the teeth.
- In most cases there is no need for surgery in the neonatal period.
- If surgery is ever needed, it is better done at 3-4 years.

Oesophageal Atresia and Tracheo-Oesophageal Fistula

- These are usually associated together.
- The incidence of oesophageal atresia is 1 in 3500 live births.
- There is usually polyhydramnios during pregnancy.
- There are 5 anatomical types, the most common of which (87%) is a blind up per oesophageal pouch and the lower part forming a vestibular communication with the trachea at its bifurcation.

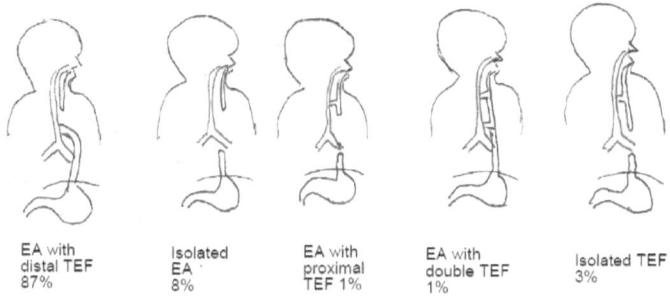

EA with distal TEF 87%   Isolated EA 8%   EA with proximal TEF 1%   EA with double TEF 1%   Isolated TEF 3%

- The first clinical sign is the accumulation of excess salivation in the mouth and pharynx with drooling. The baby requires repeated suction.
- In these cases, no feeds should be given before a wide-caliber radiopaque feeding tube is passed and checked to see if it reaches the stomach.
- If a feed is given it will result in chocking, respiratory distress with cyanosis and vomiting.
- Aspiration pneumonia may develop due to aspiration of saliva, milk or acid secretion from the stomach.

- X-ray chest should be done to see the radiopaque tube in the blind pouch. If a trachea-oesophageal fistula is present to the distal eosophagus, gas will be present in the bowel. If there is no fistula, no gas will be seen in the bowel.
- Associated anomalies that are seen in 40% of cases of Tracheo-eosophageal fistula include mainly congenital heart diseases and also intestinal anomalies. VATER Syndrome could be seen.
- Surgical correction is done either in one or more stages, depending on the abnormality, with or without gastronomy.
- Pre-operative management includes: continuous suction to drain secretions and prevent aspiration, head of the bed should be elevated to prevent gastric reflux into the lungs, IV glucose and fluids should be given and oxygen administration as needed.

Diaphragmatic Hernia

- Hernia ion of abdominal contents through a congenital defect on the diaphragm occurs in about 1 in 4000 live births.
- In most cases the hernia occurs through the posterolateral foramen of the diaphragm (foramen of Bochdalek), in 80% on the left side.
- Much less frequently, the bowel herniates through a defect in the anterolateral part of the diaphragm.
- In about 5% of cases herniation occurs through a retrosternal defect (foramen of Morgagni).
- There maybe a thin covering sac of peritorium with the herniated bowel.
- In the eventuation of the diaphragm the abdominal contents covered with a fibrous sheet bulges into the thorax and causes similar but milder symptoms.
- The clinical presentation includes:
    - Polyhydramnios
    - Scaphoid abdomen
    - Mild to severe respiratory distress at birth
    - Failure to respond to resuscitation with rapidly increasing dyspnoea or cyanosis.
    - Breath sounds in the affected hemi thorax are absent.

- In the commonest type, the heart sounds and apex beat will be displaced to the right side of the chest.
    - Bowel sounds are present on the chest.
    - Vigorous resuscitation may cause a pneumothorax in the normal lung.
    - The diagnosis is confirmed by X-ray chest and abdomen.
    - The lungs on the affected side acid also on the contra lateral side maybe hypo plastic. Pulmonary hypertension may develop.
    - Other associated anomalies include cardiac anomalies, intestinal malrotation.
- Once diaphragmatic hernia is suspected a large nasogastric tube is passed and suction is applied to prevent distension of the intrathoracic bowel.
- When the diagnosis is confirmed and signs of respiratory distress develop, endotrachial intubulation should be performed and ECMO (Exta Corporeal Membrane Oxygenation) is given.
- Surgical repair should be performed soon after stabilization.
- The high mortality rate, more than 30% is due to lung lypoplasia.

Hiatus Hernia

- This is a congenital upward protrusion of the cardiac portion of the stomach through the oesophageal hiatus in the diaphragm. It is unrelated to the acquired type of hiatus hernia of adult life. It is given the name of sliding hernia.
- The condition is not an uncommon one but it seems that some cases remain undiagnosed.
- It should be distinguished from the rare para-oesophageal hernia in which a portion of the stomach enters the chest through the hiatus but the cardiac portion of the stomach remains below the diaphragm.
- The primary cause of symptoms is free reflux of stomach contents and gastric acid up the oesophagus due to an incompetent sphincter mechanism at the cardia. This may lead to ulceration of the oesophagus followed sometimes by stricture formation.

- Clinical presentation is as follows:
  - Vomiting which is usually noted from birth. The vomitus usually contains much mucus.
  - Blood stained vomit due to oesophagitis. This is of diagnostic significance.
  - Failure to thrive early in life.
  - Iron deficiency anaemia from repeated haematemeses.
  - Positive test for occult blood in the stool.
  - The diagnosis is confirmed by barium swallow and fluoroscopy.
- Medical treatment, consisting of keeping the infant in the upright day and night and use of thickened feeds, can be successful in 70% of the patients. They become free of symptoms by the end of infancy period.
- Surgical treatment should be reserved for cases of persistent oesophagitis and when there is severe ulceration confirmed by oesophagoscopy.

Congenital Hypertrophic Pyloric Stenosis

- It is doubtful whether this relatively common disorder should be classified as congenital or as a malformation.
- The incidence is 1-8:1000 birth with male predominance. It is 1:150 in males and 1:750 in females. Risks to children of women who have had pyloric stenosis are 1:5 for sons and 1:15 for daughters. If the father was affected, the risks are 1:20 for sons and 1:40 for daughters.
- Recent studies suggests that exposure to erythromycin may lead to the development of pyloric stenosis. Also reduced tissue nitric acid levels maybe associated with development of pyloric stenosis.
- There is marked hypertrophy of the circular muscle fibers of the pylorus and severe narrowing of the pyloric canal.
- The obstruction becomes noticeable after the second week of life.
- Clinical features are:
  - Vomiting usually starts between 2 and 4 weeks, mildly at first but rapidly becomes projectile and after every feed. In 10% of cases it starts at birth.

- There is no bile in the vomitus, but may be blood stained.
- The baby is hungry and feeds greedily.
- Weight loses.
- Dehydration which may become severe enough to cause dehydration.
- Constipation as small infrequent stools.
- Visible gastric peristalsis from left to right may be seen.
- Palpation of a thickened pylorus which feels like an olive-sized mass is conclusive evidence. It is felt on deep palpation to the right of the midline especially after the child has vomited during the feed.
- The diagnosis is confirmed by ultrasound examination that shows that the thickened pylorus as a hypo echoic ring with hyper dense centre. Barium study is rarely required.
- Blood tests characteristically show hypochloremic alkalosis with potassium depletion.
- Treatment:
    - First step is to correct dehydration and electrolyte abnormality.
    - Surgical operation as Ramsted's operation or Pyloromyotomy should be performed soon after that. Results of the operation are excellent.

Congenital Duodenal Obstruction

- Congenital Duodenal Obstruction could be due to intrinsic or extrinsic causes.
- Intrinsic duodenal obstruction is caused by failure of the lumen to recanalize during the 8th to 10th week of gestational age. There could be:
    - Atresia of the duodenum, which is the most common cause of congenital duodenal obstruction. The duodenum is completely interrupted by a fibrous cord between the two segments and this is usually situated distal to ampula of vater.
    - Duodenal atresia is associated with intrauterine growth retardation or other anomalies like Down's syndrome (in

25%), a prematurity (30%). Also associated with cardiac, renal and other atresia cases.
- o Rarely, there is a web that is stretched across the lumen with a small hole in the center through which fluid can still pass.
- o Duodenal stenosis where the obstruction is not complete.
- Extrinsic duodenal obstruction could be caused by:
    - o Congenital peritoneal band.
    - o Annular pancreas which constricts the second part of the duodenum.
    - o Duodenal duplication.
    - o Malrotation of the gut.
    - o Extrinsic duodenal obstruction is rare and the obstruction caused is incomplete.
- Clinical presentation:
    - o Maternal polyhydramnios is a warning sign.
    - o Vomiting begins within a few hours after birth in the complete obstruction. It is bile-stained in most cases but in the rare cases where the atresia is above the bile duct opening, no bile will be present in the vomit.
    - o The abdomen is not distended although there may be some fullness in the epigastrium just before a vomit.
    - o Meconium may be passed normally at first.
    - o Dehydration develops rapidly.
    - o Hypochloremic metabolic alkalosis develops.
    - o Presence of these symptoms in Down's syndrome or the other associated anomalies suggests the diagnosis.
    - o Abdominal X-ray in the erect position is diagnostic. A double gas bubble is only seen, one confined to the stomach and the other to the dilated proximal duodenum. Usually fluid levels are present.
    - o When the obstruction is incomplete the symptoms develops more slowly and may suggest pyloric stenosis. The presence of bile in the vomit suggests duodenal obstruction.
    - o The presence of gas in the distal bowel on the X-ray abdomen suggests incomplete obstruction. Barium study would confirm the diagnosis.
    - o Treatment is surgical as Duodeno duodenostomy or duodeno-jejunostomy to bypass the obstruction. The

operation has a good clearance of success but the high mortality rate (35-40%) is significantly affected by the associated anomalies or prematurity.

Congenital Intestinal Obstruction below the Duodenum

- Intestinal obstruction can be caused by many congenital anomalies all of which give rise to a recognizable clinical picture consisting of:
    o Early vomiting of bile stained or brownish coloured material.
    o Distended abdomen.
    o Visible peristalsis.
    o Constipation.
    o Erect X-ray of the abdomen will show distended bowel with gases and fluid levels. The specific features will depend on underlying cause. There is a progressive dilatation cut-off at the point of obstruction.
- Causes of congenital intestinal obstruction includes:
    o Atresia of the jejunum or ileum.
    o Meconium ileus.
    o Meconium peritonitis.
    o Malrotation of the midgut.
    o Volvolus.
    o Meckel's Diverticulum.
    o Dublication of the gastrointestinal tract.
    o Herniation with strangulation of small bowel occurring through a congenital defect in the mesentry.
    o Hirschsprung's Disease.

Atresia of the Jejunum and Ileum

- This is the most common cause of intestinal obstruction. It is more frequent than duodenal atresia.
- It is probably caused by intrauterine infection.
- Antenatal ultrasound can identify the atresia.
- Polyhydramnios occurs in most affected causes.

- In two thirds of the cases, there is complete obstruction in either the distal ileum or the proximal jejunum.
- Up to 20% of the cases have multiple atresias.
- In 10% of the cases the mesentery is absent.
- Clinical presentation is classically by:
    o Repeated bile-stained vomiting within a few hours of birth.
    o Increasing abdominal distension.
    o Constipation with failure to pass meconium.
    o X-ray abdomen shows of dilated loops of small bowel and absence of colonic gas.
    o If the atresia is in the lower small bowel, a barium enema will show a narrow-caliber micro colon.
- Surgical treatment should be performed as early as possible.

Meconium Ileus

- This is mainly a presentation of cystic fibrosis (in 10-20% of cases) which is in itself a congenital anomaly as it is inherited ad autosomal recessive.
- Due to the deficiency of pancreatic enzymes the contents of the small intestine become inspissated and hence cause intestinal obstruction.
- A clue to the diagnosis is a family history of cystic fibrosis.
- The meconium is solid in nature.
- The obstruction is in the distal small bowel. It gives the same clinical presentation of bile stained vomiting, abdominal distension and constipation.
- X-ray abdomen will show dilated loops of small bowel but there will be relative absence of air-fluid levels. There may also be a finely mottled appearance of the small bowel due to small bubbles of gas trapped in the meconium filled lumen.
- Sweat chloride test should be done to confirm the diagnosis of cystic fibrosis. Positive tests show Na and Cl concentration >60mEq/L.
- Treatment is with enemas using hypertonic contrast gastrograffin media. If no improvement, surgical treatment is recommended

as enterostomy and irrigation of the intestine with saline. A temporary ileostomy may be required.

Meconium Peritonitis

- This might complicate meconium ileus or ileal atresia.
- It could be due to congenital defects in the intestinal wall.
- Non congenital causes of meconium peritonitis include necrotizing enterocolitis, which occurs mainly in premature babies, traumatic causes or drug induced (e.g. dexamethazone) or even idiopathic.
- If perforation occurred in utro, healing would be completed before birth and the infant will show no signs of intestinal obstruction at birth. There might be intra-abdominal calcification.
- When meconium peritonitis develops after birth, it will be preceded by all the signs of intestinal obstruction.
- X-ray abdomen shows gas in the peritoneal cavity with or without egg shell calcification.
- Exploratory laparotomy should be done.

Malrotation of the Gut with or Without Volvulus

- Failure to complete the normal 270 counter clockwise rotation of the intestine around the superior mesenteric artery axis, results in defective dorsal fixation of the mesentery which is also shortened.
- The bowel from the ligament of Treitz to the mid transverse colon may twist causing a volvulus around the mesenteric root thus occluding the superior mesenteric artery leading to midgut ischaemia and infarction.
- The malrotation may be associated with Ladd's bands, which are peritoneal bands running from the right posterolateral abdominal wall across the duodenum to the abnormally located caecum. They cause partial duodenal obstruction.
- Malrotation accounts for about 10% of neonatal intestinal obstruction.
- Infants present with classical symptoms of intestinal obstruction in the first 3 weeks.

- Volvulus usually occurs in the first week of life. It presents with signs of intestinal obstruction as well as shock. Bloody stools may be followed by perforation.
- Although 80% of children with malrotation and volvulus present during the neonatal period, the rest remain undetected and symptomless until later childhood or even adulthood.
- The late onset cases present with signs of intermittent intestinal obstruction, malabsorption, protein-losing enteropathy or diarrhea, or even constipation.
- 25% of symptomatic cases have associated congenital malformations, mainly cardiac.
- Abdominal X-ray shows non-specific features of small bowel obstruction.
- An upper gastrointestinal contrast media with small bowel follow through will show the abnormal position of the duodenum. Barium enema will show a mobile caecum not positioned in the right lower abdomen.
- Malrotation is repaired surgically by placing the intestine in a nonrotated position with the large bowel on the left and the small bowel on the right. Correction is by division of Ladd's bands when present. This results in widening of the base of the mesentery.
- The presence of volvulus is treated as a surgical emergency so as to present bowel necrosis.

Meckel's Diverticulum

- This is the remnant of omphalomesenteric duct. It is about 2-3cm long and is usually found on the antimesanteric border of the mid to distal ileum.
- It is the most common anomaly of the G.I. tract as it is present in 2% of the population though rarely cause symptoms. Male to female ratio is 2:1.
- The diverticulum contain, in addition to the ileal mucosa, gastric, pancreatic, jejuna or colonic mucosa. Gastric mucosa is the commonest cause of symptoms due to acid secretion and ulcerations. Symptoms occur mainly in first 2 years of life.

- Clinical presentation:
    - Painless rectal bleeding in more than half of the patients, 80% of which is Melina.
    - Intestinal obstruction as ileocolonic intussusception and volvulus occurs in 28% of patients.
    - Diverticulitis occurs in 10% of symptomatic patients usually mistaken as appendicitis.
    - Perforation and generalized peritonitis may occur.
    - The diverticulum may be trapped in an inguinal hernia (Littre Hernia).
    - Chronic recurrent abdominal pain could be the only symptom.
- Diagnosis of Meckel's diverticulum is not made by barium study. To detect ectopic gastric mucosa in a bleeding Meckel's diverticulum is by using nuclear scintigraphy. A well defined focal accumulation of radio nuclide usually appears at or about the same time as activity in the stomach and gradually increases in intensity. When the site of bleeding is not clear, angiography may be useful.
- Treatment is by surgical resection.

Duplication of the Gastrointestinal Tract

- Duplications are congenital anomalies that can occur anywhere from the mouth to the anus but most commonly in the ileum.
- Most duplications do not communicate with the intestinal lumen but are attached to the mesenteric side of the gut.
- Some duplications are neuroenteric cysts as they are attached to the spinal cord and are associated with hemi vertebrae and spina bifida.
- In the abdomen they become gradually filled with secretions (fluid) and compress the adjacent normal bowel causing intestinal obstruction. They produce a palpable abdominal mass.
- Clinical presentation that may occur from infancy period include:
    - Features of intestinal obstruction.
    - Colicky abdominal pain.
    - Rectal bleeding.

- o Diarrhea and malabsorption due to bacterial overgrowth in the communicating duplications.
- X-ray abdomen shows a non calcified mass displacing the intestine. Nuclear Scintigraphy will detect the presence of gastric mucosa, if any.
- Treatment is by surgical resection.

Hirschsprung Disease

- This is due to the absence of ganglion cells in the mucosal and muscular layers of the colon. It is limited to the recto sigmoid colon in 75% of cases but the entire colon is aganglionic in 8% of patients. It is almost entirely a disease of males.
- There is a failure of relaxation of the affected bowel, abscent peristalsis and obstruction to the passage of faeces. The intestine proximal to the aganglionic segment becomes dilated and its mucosa may become thin and inflamed resulting in diarrhea, bleeding and protein loss.
- The commonest presentation is neonatal intestinal obstruction, with failure to pass meconium. It accounts for one fifth of cases of neonatal intestinal obstruction.
- It might present after the neonatal period with severe constipation and failure to thrive. The stools are offensive and ribbon-like. Iron deficiency anaemia and hypoproteinaemia are seen.
- P/R examination reveals an empty anal canal and rectum despite faecal impaction felt on abdominal examination and on x-ray examination. If it is a short segment Hirschsprug's disease there may be a gush of flatus and stool as the figure is withdrawn.
- Hirschsprug's disease is relatively more common in association with Down's syndrome and Waardenburg Syndrome. There is a family history in 5% cases.
- X-ray abdomen may reveal multiple dilated loops of bowel with air-fluid levels consistent with a distal obstruction. There is absence of rectal gas and the rectal diameter is smaller than colonic diameter.
- Barium enema will show a narrow segment distally with a proximal dilated colon.

- Rectal biopsy is diagnostic as well as it will reveal the length of the aganglionic segment.
- Treatment is surgical done in two stages. The first stage is to perform a colostomy proximal to the aganglionic segment. This is better delayed until the age of 3 months. Meanwhile, the baby can have repeated saline rectal washouts. In the second stage, resection of the aganglionic segment is done and a surgical pull-through of ganglionatted bowel to the pre-anal rectal remnant is made. The second stage is done when the infant is at least 6 months of age.
- Complications following surgery are rare. They include chronic constipation, due to anal stenosis, faecal incontinence and anastomosis stricture or breakdown.

Congenital Anorectal Malformation

- These occur once in every 4000-5000 births. They are detected by careful inspection of perianal area at birth.
- They include:
    o Anterior displacement of anus.
    o Anal stenosis.
    o Imperforate anal membrane.
    o Anal agenesis (about 10% of the cases).
    o Anorectal agenesis (about 75% of the cases). There is fistula formation in most cases.
    o Rectal atresia.
- About half of these cases are associated with vertebral or genitourinary malformation.
- Most types are more common in males except the anterior displacement of the anus which is more common in girls.
- Anal stenosis is usually treated with simple dilatation but other anomalies are treated surgically.

Abdominal Wall Malformations

- The defects in the abdominal wall includes:
    o Umbilical Hernia

- o Omphalocele
- o Gastroschitis

Umbilical Hernia

- This is the result of incomplete closure of the fascia of the umbilical ring.
- The herniated omentum or bowel is covered by skin.
- It is commonly seen in premature infants or African babies.
- Most umbilical hernia regresses spontaneously if the facial defect is less than 1.5cm in diameter. Surgical reduction of the hernia and closure of the defect is done if the defect has a diameter of more than 1.5cm by the age of two years, or if small bowel has incarcerated.
- Reducing the hernia and strapping the skin by a coin does not accelerate the healing process. It only makes parents not visualizing large hernia.
- Para umbilical hernia does not regress spontaneously.

Omphalocele

- This is herniation of abdominal contents including liver and spleen into the umbilical stalk itself so that the cord is inserted into part of the hernia sac which is covered by amniotic membrane and peritoneum.
- The incidence of omphalocele is 1:6000 births. 10% of cases are prematures.
- The thin covering layer might rupture during delivery.
- There is a high incidence of associated anomalies, namely gastrointestinal defects in 1/3 of the cases, cardiac defects in ¼ of cases and Beckwith Syndrome in 10% of the cases and trisomy 13.
- Management of Omphalocele includes:
    - o Covering the defect with a sterile dressing soaked with warm saline.
    - o Nasogastric tubes for suction and decompression.
    - o I.V. fluids and glucose with I.V. antibiotics.

- o Surgical treatment with primary closure for small defects. For large defects, a staged closure is performed with gradual reduction of the abdominal contents into the abdominal cavity after covering it with a prosthetic material and a secondary closure.

Gastroschisis

- This is herniation of the intestine through an abdominal wall defect lateral to the umbilical cord, usually on its right.
- There is no covering sac, no membrane and no liver or spleen outside the abdomen.
- Few cases are associated with intestinal atresia but up to 60% of the cases are born prematurely.
- The surgical treatment is the same as Omphalocele.

Inguinal Hernia

- A peritoneal sac precedes the testicle as it descends, during the fetal development, from the genital ridge to the scrotum. The lower portion of this sac envelops the testis to form the tunica vaginalis while the remainder atrophies just before birth.
- If this sac (the processus vaginalis) remains open as it might happen in 50% of the cases, peritoneal fluid or abdominal contents may be forced into it to form an indirect inguinal hernia.
- Most inguinal hernias are of the indirect type and occur commonly in premature infants.
- Male to female incidence is 9:1 and are mostly right sided.
- Hernias may be present at birth or may appear at any time later, as painless swelling in the inguinal area. The hernia may retract and a history of inguinal fullness is often the only diagnostic clue.
- The contents of the hernia can be reduced easily with gentle pressure.
- Sometimes a loop of intestine may become partially or completely obstructed leading to intestinal obstruction. This will lead to

incarcerated hernia which will require immediate surgery to prevent bowel or testicular necrosis.
- A symptomatic reducible hernia should be repaired surgically as soon as possible.

Intestinal Polyps

- Juvenile Polyps are the most common type and in 80% of cases occur in the recto sigmoid colon. They are benign and are usually solitary preduncilated hamartoms. There is usually a positive family history. None malignant.
- Juvenile polyps present between 2-6 years with painless blood per rectum. They are more frequent in boys. They do not cause abdominal pain but could be a lead point for an intussusception. They may be palpated on P/R examination.
- Colonoscopy is both diagnostic and therapeutic as the polyp can be removed at the same time.

Familial Polyposis of the Colon

- Inherited as autosomal dominant with high incidence of intestinal carcinoma.
- Children of affected adults must come under suspicion as having 50:50 chance of developing the disease.
- Polyps are usually multiple and may reach hundreds in numbers. They are hyper plastic with focal adenomatous change.
- Diarrhea is a common early symptom.
- The only treatment is early and total colectomy. The rectum may be preserved if free of polyps.

Peutz-Jeghers Syndrome

- Inherited as autosomal dominant. It is not premalignant with incidence of less than 2%.

- The polyps are in the upper intestine, involving the jejunum, duodenum and sometimes even the stomach. The polyps are multiple hamartomas.
- There are mucocutaneous pigmentations that look like freckles and are characteristically distributed on the lips, buccal mucous membranes, face, palms and soles.
- There may be associated ovarian cysts and tumors.
- Abdominal symptoms vary from attacks of incomplete intestinal obstruction due to recurrent intussusceptions to frank melena and hematemesis.
- Diagnosis is confirmed by barium meal.
- Treatment is by surgical removal of accessible polyps or those causing obstruction and bleeding.

Gardner Syndrome

- It is inherited as autosomal dominant. It is highly malignant. The polyps are located mainly in the colon but may be in the intestine and stomach.
- There are multiple polyps and adenomatous.
- There are soft tissue and bone tumors as part of the syndrome. Retinal pigmentation may be present.
- Treatment is by total colactomy.

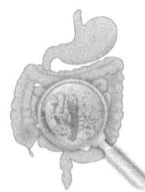

FUNCTIONAL GASTRO-INTESTINAL DISORDERS DURING INFANCY

Physiology

- o The intestinal surface area is the largest of the body measuring about 3000 m2, approximately the area of a tennis court. It hosts about 70% of the human body immune cells.
- o The gut function and the microbiota development have a great impact on the development of:
    * The digestion and absorption of nutrients and vitamin production, hence promotes growth.
    * The immune system and defense against viral and bacterial pathogens.
    * Nervous system development with impact on mood, behavior and overall wellbeing.
- o The development of the microbial colonization of the infant gut occurs after birth and has been associated with important health and disease issues. It is dependent on many factors including host genetics, mode of deliver, method of feeding whether breast or formula feeding, diet, antibiotics use and the environment.
- o Human milk is thought to be an important source of bacteria that may help to colonize the infant gut and so contributes to the composition of its micro biota.

Functional Gastro-intestinal Disorders (FGIDs)

- o FGIDs are very common in children of all ages but more significant among infants across the globes with estimated global incidence ranging from 40-60% thus affecting about half the population of infants. They comprise a range of chronic or / and recurrent disorders that are the result of abnormal functioning of gastrointestinal tract but cannot be explained by anatomical, structural or biochemical abnormalities.
- o FGIDs occur in otherwise healthy infants and are diagnosed according to the symptom-based. These mainly include: infant regurgitation, colic, constipation, and functional diarrhea. Other less common occurring include: infant dyschezia, infant rumination, and cyclic infant vomiting.
- o FGIDs tend to resolve as the infant grows, but they can be very disruptive for families causing significant distress and anxiety. They may reduce the quality of parent infant interaction and are associated with maternal postpartum depressive symptoms and premature discontinuation of breast feeding. They also drain precious health resources.
- o It can be challenging to distinguish between functional digestive symptoms, which should naturally resolve over time, and symptoms caused by underlying medical condition that might require special treatment.

Infant Regurgitation

- o Infant regurgitation is the most common FGID in infancy. It is defined as the passage of stomach contents up the pharynx into the mouth. It is not the same as vomiting which is defined as central nervous system reflex involving both voluntary and
- o involuntary muscle. Gastroesophageal reflux (GER) episodes occur when stomach contents move backward up into the esophagus. GER is part of regurgitation and many healthy newborns and infants experience it. It is different from GERD, gastroesophageal reflux disease, where GER leads to complications or contributes to tissue damage or inflammation hence causing troublesome

- symptoms like persistent crying, irritability, back arching and sleeping problems.
o According to Rome iii/iv criteria a diagnosis of infant regurgitation happens when the infant experiences regurgitation episodes at least twice a day for at least 3 weeks in the absence of symptoms of abnormal posture, difficulty feeding or swallowing, difficulty of breathing, aspiration, apnoea, failure of thrive, haematemesis or passing blood in stools, persistent vomiting, diarrhoea, constipation, abdominal distension, seizures or any suspected genetic abnormality.
o At its peak age around 2-4 months the prevalence rates of infant regurgitation has been reported to be as 67-87%. Factors that contribute to the high incidence include: infant lying down lat most of the time, almost completely fluid diet, immature lower esophagus sphincter, over feeding and premature delivery.
o Infant regurgitation is a self-limiting and benign condition that tends to decrease significantly by 1 year of age in most healthy infants. Nevertheless it can cause considerable stress in the family.
o Management of infant regurgitation include:
  * The most important part of treatment is parental reassurance and education about feeding particularly with respect to avoidance of overfeeding, feeding frequently and correct feeding technique.
  * Monitoring of infant growth ad weight gain.
  * Give the baby smaller and frequent feeds.
  * Feed the baby in upright position and hold the baby upright in sitting position for 20-30 minutes after feeding.
  * Frequent burps during and after feeding to get rid of swallowed air.
  * Change the size of the nipple on the baby bottle as too large or too small nipple can cause the baby to swallow air.
  * Thickening formula: either by use of anti-regurgitation formula or expected breast milk thickened with rice cereals, corn or potato starch.
  * Use of anti-regurgitation bed with an elevated head angle at 45 degrees has been recommended by some with doubtful positive results.

* Consider food allergy diagnosis especially cow's milk protein allergy (CMPA) in infants who have atopic dermatitis or wheezing. CMPA is managed by trial elimination and reintroduction. Breast fed mothers are advised to take cow's milk-free diet and formula fed infants to use extensively hydrolysed formula.

Functional Constipation

- o Bowel movement frequently varies from more than 4 stools per day during the first week after birth to about 2 stools per day at 2 years of age and around 1 stool per day at 4 years of age.
- o Constipation is generally defined as difficult and / or rare defecation < one stool per week in breastfed and < one stool per 3 days in formula fed infants, lasting for at least 2 weeks.
- o The Rome iii criteria define functional constipation in early life up to 4 years of age as fulfilling at least 2 of the following criteria for at least one month:
    * Two or fewer defecation per week.
    * History of excessive stool retention.
    * History of painful or hard bowel movement.
    * Presence of a large faecal mass in the rectum.
    * History of large diameter stool.
- o In toilet trained children the following additional criteria may be used:
    * At least one episode per week of incontinence after acquisition of toilet skills.
    * History of large diameter stool which obstruct the toilet.
- o Functional constipation constitutes 95% of infant constipation. The prevalence varies from study to another but in average it is 15-20%.
- o Only 5% of infantile constipation may be due to organic causes, the most common of which is cow's milk protein allergy, Hirschsprung disease and cystic fibrosis.
- o The red flag for possible organic disease include:
    * Presentation during the neonatal period.

- * Absence of meconium within the first 36 hours of life in a term infant.
- * Bloody stools, not due to anal fissure.
- * Failure to thrive and/or signs of systemic illness on physical examination like anal or sacral abnormalities or neurodevelopment delay.
- * Vomiting especially bilious vomiting.
- o Diagnosis of functional infantile constipation is done on:

A/ History, ask for:
- * Passage of meconium within the first 36 hours of life in a term baby. Preterm babies usually pass meconium later. Causes of delayed passage of meconium include: Hirschsprung's disease, meconium ileus in cystic fibrosis, intestinal obstruction, small left colon, functional ileus and maternal drugs.
- * Family history of severe atopic dermatitis.
- * Feeding history.
- * Any associated symptoms.

B/ Physical examination which should include:
- * General examination looking for evidence of failure to thrive, severe atopic dermatitis, and signs of hypothyroidism.
- * Abdominal examination looking for distension, masses, faecal impaction.
- * Anal and per anal examination looking for anal tone, fissures and anal cracks, scars, perianal sensation and reflex.
- * Back and spine for pigmentation, dimples, tufts for hair over lumbosacral region, sacral agenesis and dysraphism.
- * Neurological examination for sensory or motor defects of the lower extremities, hypotonia and neuropathic conditions.

C/ In the absence of red flags, the diagnosis is functional constipation. No need for blood tests, no need for abdominal x-rays or ultrasound, no need for barium enema or anorectal manometer.

D/ Anal stimulation is not recommended.

- Management
    * Early diagnosis and early management is important as delayed management for more than three months might lead to life time constipation.
    * Hard stools might lead to painful defecation that will lead to voluntary withholding of faeces causing prolonged stasis in the colon & reabsorption of fluids leading to harder stools and hence more painful defecation, it becomes a vicious circle.
    * Prolonged constipation is associated with social withdrawal, loss of self-esteem, depressive behavior and reduce quality of life in children beyond infancy period.
    * The first step in the management of functional constipation is reassurance of the parents of its benign nature. Drugs used in treatment are:
        - Lactulose used for infants less than 6 months of age in a dose 1-2 gm/kg (1-3ml/kg) once or twice a day.
        - Macrogol (Polyethyllene glycol –PEG) in infants above 6 months of age, in a dose of 1-1.5 gm/kg/day for 3 days.
        - Milk of magnesia, dose for 2-5 years is 400mg to 1200 mg/day orally for 7 days. It can be used together with fiber diet (fruits and vegetables) and probiotics.
        - Probiotics, namely Lactobacillus Reuteri (BioGaia) and BififobacteriumLongum (Co-PRO) are the ones used 5b drops/day for 10 days.
        - Prebiotic oligosaccharides, in combination with other ingredients such as beta-palmitate and partial protein hydrolysates soften the stools in constipated infants.
        - There is evidence of some benefit using partially hydrolysed infant formula with prebiotics (GOS/FOS) and beta-palmitate for constipation in formula fed infants.
        - Rectal disimpaction should only used for acute relief.
        - Laxatives should be continued for 1-3 months. Most important is to start toilet training immediately if it has not been applied before.

Infantile colic

- All babies cry when they are hungry, wet, cold, hot or tired. However infantile colic is defined as episodes of crying for more than 3 hours a day, for more than 3 days a week in the preceding week, in an otherwise healthy baby and with no clear cause. It usually starts a few weeks after birth with a peak at around 6 weeks but stops by 4 month of age. It affects 10-30% of infants and occurs equally in boys & girls, breast fed & formula fed.
- The crying often occurs in the late afternoon or evening. It is intense and often high pitched. When crying the baby's face is red & flushed with wrinkled brows, fists clenched, arms and legs bend toward the abdomen and having tensed abdominal muscles. The baby may pass wind during crying. It is extremely difficult to comfort the baby during the episode. This can be very distressing, exhausting and emotionally draining for the parents or caregiver.
- Babies with infantile colic are fine between the episodes. They feed well, grow well and do not show any other sign of illness. Nevertheless, infant colic is associated with parental anxiety, postpartum depression, disruption of parents relationship and family routine, early termination of breast feeding, tempting to overfeeding, reducing face to face interaction with the infant and increased risk of of child abuse especially shaken baby syndrome. It is also associated with frequent visits to doctors, excessive laboratory tests and prescription of medications as well as loss of parental work time.
- Less than 5% of infants with excess crying have an underlying organic disease. The warning symptoms and signs indicating further assessment and investigations to exclude an organic disease include: poor sucking, drinking less milk than usual, fever, vomiting, constipation, diarrhoea especially with blood and mucous, irritability or lethargy and being more sleepy than usual, change in breathing rate or effort or grunting, failure to thrive, seizures and the presence of severe atopic dermatitis.
- The exact cause of infantile colic is not known but researchers have explored a number of possibilities:
    * Immaturity of the central nervous system with disbalance of the pathway leading to unstable cyclic behaviour, infantile migraine or subdural haemorrhage.

- * Psychological causes like parental anxiety and inadequate infant-family relationship, or the baby is still adjusting to the surrounding of loud noise, light etc.
- * Change in the level of hormones that control the movement of the gut muscles leading to muscle spasm or fussy mood and oversensitivity to gas in the intestine.
- * Food allergy or intolerance to items in the mother's diet, most commonly is cow's milk protein. Exclusion of cow's milk protein from the maternal diet or use of extensively hydrolysed infant formula in formula fed infants has been beneficial in decreasing infantile colic in some infants. Lactose intolerance is suspected in some cases especially post gastroenteritis.
- * Abnormal balance of bacteria in the gut may affect gastrointestinal development and gut motility with gas production leading to colic. Some studies have shown that difference in the composition of Lactobacillus species in the gut may cause infantile colic.
- * Constipation, GER, anal fissure, eczema & severe nappy rash, and a foreign body in the eye or corneal laceration may be an underlying cause to the crying.
- * Smoking during pregnancy does increase the risk of the baby developing infantile colic, also passive smoking increases the risk.
- o Diagnosis of infantile colic is by exclusion of other causes of crying. This is properly done through detailed history and physical examination searching for any of the above mentioned warning symptoms signs. It is important to exclude surgical emergency conditions namely intestinal obstruction e.g. volvulus, intussusceptions, strangulated hernia or twisted testicle. Infections like urinary tract infection, ear infection, appendicitis and meningitis should be excluded as well as none accidental injuries. In most cases these conditions can be excluded by history and physical examination with no need to perform tests such as blood tests and x-rays.
- o Management:
  - * The most important step is reassurance of parents that infantile colic is a benign condition that typically resolves spontaneously by 3-4 months of age. Parents should also be

told that colic is not a result of poor parenting and does not mean that the baby is rejecting them. They should be advised to create a positive atmosphere. Extra support for them may be useful. Breastfeeding mothers should be encouraged to continue breastfeeding.
* There is no treatment that cures colic. Calming measures may be helpful in some babies. These measures include: soothing by holding the baby during a crying episode, holding the baby upright during feeding to prevent the baby swallowing air and burping the baby in between and after feeding, feed smaller amounts more frequently, breastfeeding or using pacifier, rocking the baby gently while supporting the head but never shaking the baby, giving the baby a warn bath or gentle massage of the baby's belly. Some people say white noise in the background like noise made by washing machine, vacuum cleaner or a moving car engine help to soothe the colicky baby.
* If cow's milk protein allergy is suspected, then the use of extensively hydrolysed infant formula in a formula fed infant and a cow's milk free diet for a breastfeeding mother may be beneficial to decrease infant colic. However if the baby's symptoms do not improve after 1 week of cow's milk elimination, then babies should return to their normal feed.
* In formula fed infants consider feeding with partial protein hydrolysed formula with added beta-palmitate and prebiotic mixture of short chain galacto-oligosaccharide (scGOS) and long chain fructo-oligosaccharide (lsFOS), when CMPA is not suspected. Some data suggests this may be beneficial in reducing infant colic.
* In breastfed infants consider treatment with the probiotic Lactobacillus reuteri(Bio Gaia) drops as some reports suggest it reduces infant colic in breastfed infants but not formula fed infants. Breastfeeding mothers should avoid too much caffeine in their diet.
* Medicines: There is no firm evidence that any of the drugs are beneficial. Medicines that have been tried include: Simethicone which is safe but does not appear to work, Dicyclomine works in some babies but is not without side effects, Cimetropium bromide has no evidence to support its

use. Alternative medicines like Herbal teas, Gripe water and Homeopathic remedies have been used but with little evidence of their benefit.

Functional diarrhea

- Functional diarrhoea is the diarrhoea that occurs in otherwise healthy infants who are normally active and growing with no evidence of systemic disease, infection, malnutrition or malabsorption. The diagnosis of functional diarrhoea in infants and toddlers by Rome IV criteria requires all of the following:
    * Daily recurrent passage of 4 or more large painless unformed stools.
    * Symptoms lasting more than 4 weeks.
    * Onset of symptoms that begin between 6 and 60 months of age.
    * Passage of stools that occur during waking hours.
    * No failure to thrive where caloric intake is adequate.
- Toddlers diarrhea is the same as functional diarrhea. Dietary factors such as overfeeding, excessive fruit juice composition, excessive carbohydrate ingestion especially fructose with low fat intake, low fiber diet and excessive sorbitol intake are underlying causes.
- Diagnosis is made through:
    * Proper history taking enquiring about diet history of overfeeding, excessive fruit juice or sorbitol consumption, excessive carbohydrate ingestion with low fat intake, any food allergy, any recent enteric infection, use of laxatives, antibiotics or diet change.
    * Physical examination to show that the child is growing normally and has no underlying pathology. Stool examination may be done to exclude evidence of infection, inflammation, blood in stools and to reassure parents of the benign nature of the condition. It is important to avoid unnecessary tests but not at the expense of missing an organic treatable cause of chronic diarrhoea.

- o   Treatment is mainly based on reassurance of parents that the condition is not harmful and is self limiting, as well as advising them to correct any underlying dietary cause.

Dyschezia

- o   Dyschezia is a functional condition characterized by straining, screaming, crying, and turning red on the face while making an effort to defecate in an infant that has daily soft stools. These symptoms continue for 10-20 minutes which can be distressing for the infant and parent. These episodes can happen many times each day. The cause is thought to be related to failure to coordinate increased intra abdominal pressure with relaxation of the pelvic muscles. The straining and crying may be associated with both successful and unsuccessful passage of the soft stools. It is not constipation. In Rome IV the age limit is 1-9 months of age.
- o   The anxiety caused by these episodes may prompt parents to visit doctors during the infant 2-3 months of age with concerns that their infant is constipated. The crying is not due to pain but is the infant's attempt to create intra abdominal pressure before they learn to bear down more effectively for bowel movement.
- o   Diagnosis: history will reveal normal diet, normal sleeping, normal weight gain and normal growth. Though, physical examination should be performed in the presence of parents so they are reassured that nothing abnormal was missed. The examination will show normal growth and no abnormality detected. Stool examination is normal.
- o   Treatment: reassurance is the major step in the management, as the condition will resolve spontaneously. Parents are advised to avoid rectal stimulation as this may be disturbing to the infant or may condition the infant to wait for stimulation to defecate. No need for use of laxatives.

Rumination syndrome

- o Rumination is a functional disorder in which the infant habitually and voluntarily regurgitates stomach contents back into the oral cavity and re-chews partially digested food that has already been swallowed. In most cases the re-chewed food is then swallowed again, but rarely the child spit it out. This disorder occurs in children who had previously been eating normally. It typically happens daily during feeding or right after feeding. It is seen in all age groups but mostly occurs in infants and young children between 3-8 months and in children with intellectual disabilities.
- o There is repetitive contraction of the abdominal muscles, diaphragm and tongue. This leads to the regurgitation of the gastric contents into the mouth. Symptoms result from the way the brain and the digestive system are interacting.
- o Causes: The exact cause of rumination is not known but several factors that may contribute to its development were suggested (Web MD):
    * Triggering events e.g. viral infections, GI disease or change in the patient life causing stress. These triggering events can make having food or liquid in the stomach uncomfortable, hence the body learned to contract the abdominal muscles resulting in regurgitation. After the triggering event has gone away the regurgitation behaviour remains in the place and becomes as a habit.
    * Neglect of or an abnormal relationship between the child and the mother may cause child to engage in self-comfort by the act of chewing.
    * It may a way for the child to gain attention.
    * It may be a manifestation of mental illness such as depression or anxiety.
- o Diagnosis of rumination is by detailed history and physical examination. For diagnosis the following should be fulfilled:
    * At least 2 months history of repeated regurgitation and re-chewing or expulsion of food
    * The behavior begins soon after ingestion of a meal.
    * The behavior does not occur during sleep.
    * No retching.

- - * No evidence of organic disease.
    * Symptom does not respond to standard treatment of GERD.
  - o Treatment: There is no specific treatment for rumination. The management aims at changing the child's behavior through:
    * Changing the child's posture during and immediately after eating
    * Encouraging more interaction between child and mother during feeding, giving the child more attention.
    * Reducing distraction during feeding.
    * Make feeding a more relaxing and pleasurable experience.
    * Distracting the child when begins the rumination behavior.
    * Blood test for anemia and electrolyte imbalance to treat any abnormality caused.
    * Nutritional rehabilitation in case malnutrition has developed as a result of rumination.
  - o Complications of untreated rumination include:
    * Malnutrition.
    * Failure to thrive and weight loss.
    * Dehydration.
    * Stomach disease such as ulcer.
    * Bad breath and tooth decay.

Cyclic Vomiting Syndrome (CVS)

- o 2% of children suffer episodes of vomiting, at least, 5 times a year, younger children are more affected than older children.
- o Cyclic vomiting occurs from infancy to middle- age adulthood with a peak prevalence between 2 and 7 years.
- o CVS is a stereotypic, recurrent episodes of vomiting which last from hours to few days with symptom- free interval periods which last weeks to months. The vomiting should not be attributed to another disorder that cause vomiting.
- o Vomiting may occur sporadically or at regular intervals and are characterized by onset at the same time of the day, most often late at night or early in the morning. However, these may be different from patient to patient.

- Other symptoms that are associated with CVS include: nausea and retching, lack of appetite and lack of sleep, sensitivity to light, abdominal pain with or without diarrhea, pallor, fatigue and not wanting to talk, thirst, headache and low grade fever.
- There is no known cause for CVS but there are some triggering factors which include:
    * Respiratory infections or sinus infections.
    * Emotional stress.
    * Reaction to some foods like chocolate, cheese, caffeine.
    * Change of season or very hot weather.
    * Overeating or eating immediately before bedtime and fasting.
    * Physical exhaustion and sleep deprivation.
    * Periods in young females.
    * Motion sickness.
- The diagnosis is through detailed history and physical examination. Blood tests, urine examination, x-ray and ultrasound scan may be needed to exclude organic cause.
- Management:
    * During the attack stay in bed in quiet dark room, take small sips of fluids to prevent dehydration.
    * After the vomiting attack has finished drink plenty of fluids and gradually resume normal diet.
    * Avoid known triggers, getting enough sleep, try to manage stress and anxiety and eating small carbohydrate- based snacks between meals, before exercise and at bed time.
- Treatment focus on 2 aspects of CVS attacks, not for children less than 12 years:
    1. Prevention of the episode: daily treatment with cyproheptadine, pizotifen, amitriptyline, propranolol or erythromycin can diminish the frequency of the episodes or can even prevent them entirely.
    2. Reduce the severity of the attacks: Oral acid-inhibiting drugs for the protection of the esophagus mucosa and Lorazepam for antiemetic, anxiolytic and sedative purposes can be considered.

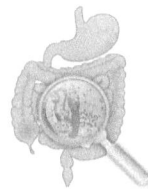

ACQUIRED GASTROINTESTINAL DISORDERS

Acute Stomatitis

This is infection and inflammation of the oral cavity. The causes are:

1. Aphthous ulcer is the most common infectious lesion in the oral cavity.
    a. The ulcers are often recurrent and may appear singly or confluent.
    b. The exact aetiology of aphthous ulcers is not known but it is believed to be infectious or due to allergic or autoimmune manifestations.
    c. The ulcers are found on the insides of the lips or in the interior mouth.
    d. They may be painful and last for 1-2 weeks. There is no associated fever.
    e. Treatment is by coating the lesion with betamethasone valerate ointment or kenalogy in orabase
2. Herpes Simplex is the most common viral infection to cause gingivostomatitis which can be very severe at times.
    a. In many cases the primary infection is subclinical.
    b. In severe cases the child is ill with high fever, pain in the mouth, anorexic and unable to eat or drink. There will be tender cervical lymph nodes.
    c. The gingivostomatitis last for 7-10 days.

d. Treatment is symptomatic. Steroids are contra indicated. Acyclovir suspension should be started early in a dose of 20mg/kg/dose, 4 times/day x 5 days.
   e. I.V. fluids should be given to dehydrated children.
3. Coxsachie virus infection (Herpangina) is a less common cause of stomatitis.
   a. It causes severe ulcerative lesions on the posterior part of the mouth.
   b. The initial lesions are vesicular than ulcerations and plaques follow.
   c. High fever, malaise and toxaemia may develop with feeding difficulties.
   d. The condition is self limited and the treatment is symptomatic. Topical analgesics like 2% viscous xylocaine could be used.
   e. Some Coxachicvirus may involve may involve the hand and feet at the same time with the mouth (Hand-Mouth-Foot Syndrome).
4. Candida albicans infection (Thrush)
   a. It usually appears as white patches with surrounding inflammation on the oral mucosa.
   b. It is seen in infants, immunosuppressed patients and patients on antibiotics.
   c. Patients with diabetes mellitus are especially prone to Candida infection.
   d. Inhalation of steroids for Asthma predisposes patients to thrush.
   e. HIV infection should be considered if there is no other reason for oral thrush.
   f. Treatment is by Nystatin 200,000 units 4 times daily.
5. Behcet Disease
   a. This is a rare disorder which includes recurrent aphthous stomatitis, genital ulceration and iritis. Arthritis is a major problem and is usually pauciarticular.

b. Skin lesions with erythema multiform and erythema nodosum could be seen with the arthritis.
c. Treatment includes oral steroids.
6. FAPA Syndrome (Fever, Aphthus, Stomatitis, Pharyngitis and Cervical Adenopathy)
   a. This syndrome was first described in 1987.
   b. The cause is not known, but it is believed to be an inflammatory condition.
   c. It is a recurrent condition which recurs every 4-6 weeks.
   d. It affects children before the age of 5 years and continuous through adolescence, after which it resolves spontaneously.
   e. The condition improves with prednisolone and may resolve with tonselectomy. The ulcers respond well to betamethasome valerate.
7. Familial Mediterranean Fever
   a. This is an uncommon familial disorder with an autosomal recessive inheritance pattern.
   b. It is characterized by acute recurrent attacks of fever, peritonitis, pleuritis or synovitis and arthritis. There might be oedema of the tongue and erythema of buccal mucosa.
   c. The fever lasts 24 to 48 hours.
   d. Analgesics and antipyretics will help in the acute attacks. Colchicines has been used a prophylactic drug for severe cases.

Gastroesophageal Reflux Disease

- It refers to passage of gastric contents into the esophagus. It is a common problem.
- Factors that lead to GERD includes:
    o Reduced lower esophagus sphincter pressure.
    o Poor esophageal contraction.
    o Gastric detention.
    o Delayed gastric emptying for any reason.
    o Hiatus hernia if large.
    o Transient relaxation of the lower esophageal sphincter.

- Presentation of gastroesophageal reflux could typically be:
    - Excessive regurgitation is the most common symptom.
    - Vomiting.
    - Failure to thrive.
    - Irritability.
    - Choking and dysphagia.
    - Epigastric/chest pain in older children due to esophagitis.
    - Colic after feeding.
    - Haematemesis.
    - Occult or gross blood in stools.
    - Sandifer Syndrome with the infant manifesting lateral head tilt and back arching due to esophagitis.
    - Esophageal obstruction due to esophageal stricture.
    - Aspiration pneumonia.
    - Iron deficiency anaemia
- Gastroesophageal reflux disease could have the following atypical presentation.
    - Chronic cough.
    - Wheezing and asthma-like attacks.
    - Apnoea and bradycardia.
    - Excessive hiccups.
    - Sleep disturbance.
    - Rumination.
- Diagnosis of gastroesophageal reflux disease is mainly a clinical one. A detailed history will help in reaching the diagnosis in the mild cases. When severe symptoms develop due to esophagitis, the following tests are done:
    - Baruim Swallow with fluoroscopy. This will diagnose large hiatus hernia or any obstructive cause. Free regurgitate can also be observed.
    - Esophageal pH probe study for 24 hours is the definitive test to establish the reflux. It shows the period of time the esophageal pH is less than 4.0.
    - If the % of time pH less than 4 is 5-10% it is mild reflux, if it is 10-20% this is moderate reflux and if it is more than 20% the reflux is a severe one. The normal esophageal pH is considered to be close to pH 7.0.

- o Esophageal manometry can be done to measure the lower esophageal sphincter pressure.
- o Esophageal and gastric scintiscanning using Tc 99m can be used in indentifying pulmonary aspiration.
- o Esophagoscopy will identify esophagitis.
- Management of Gastroesophageal Reflux Disease
  - o In about 80% of the cases the symptoms are self limited disappearing in infants between 6 months and 12 months of age. This is due to introduction of solid feeding and infants obtaining the erect position by sitting.
  - o Mild to moderate cases are managed by:
    - Feeding the infant with small frequent feeds.
    - Thickening the feeds with rice cereals.
    - Use anti reflux milk.
    - Placing the infant after feeds in a 45 degree upright position may provide an element of gravity in preventing reflux of gastric contents.
    - Reassurance to parents after full explanation of the condition.
  - o Severe cases complicated by esophagitis are treated and managed by:
    - H2 blocking agents like Ranitidine, 5mg/kg/day in two divided doses.
    - Proton pump inhibitors like Omeprazole.
    - These two helps in reducing acid reflux.
    - Metoclopramide, 0.1mg/kg before meals increases gastric emptying and improves esophageal motor function.
    - Bethanechol which is a parasympathomimetic agent increases esophageal peristalsis and lower esophageal sphincter tone.
  - o Resistent cases will require surgical treatment, the most common operation being Nissen Fundoplication. Here, the fundus of the stomach is wrapped 270-360 degree around the distal esophagus. Indication for surgery include:
    - ➢ Persistent vomiting with failure to thrive.
    - ➢ Recurrent esophagitis or esophageal stricture.
    - ➢ Repeated attacks of aspiration pneumonia.

> Severe apnoea attacks.
> Failure to respond to 6 weeks of medical treatment.

Achalasia of the Esophagus *see page 49 for details.*

Peptic Ulcer

- Inflammation of the gastric mucosa (gastritis) and duodenal mucosa (duodinitis) can occur without the formation of ulcer.
- Helicobacter pylori is the most common cause of duodenal ulcers in children as well as it causes chronic gastritis (detected in 90% of duodenal ulcers and 70% of gastric ulcers).
- Other causes of ulcers in childhood includes:
    o Anti inflammatory drugs (Asprin and NSAIDS) which reduce mucosal protective mechanisms.
    o Conditions that cause reduced metabolic activity of the mucosal cells, such as hypotension and hypoxia.
    o Conditions that cause increased secretion of acid or pepsin as in increased parietal cell mass and increased vagal tone.
    o Reflux of bile from duodenum to stomach.
    o Conditions in which there is decreased neutralizing activity in duodenal secretions.
    o Zollinger-Ellison Syndrome where there are multiple gastric and duodenal ulcers due to gastric producing tumor of the endocrine pancreas.
    o Crohn's Disease, hepatic Cirrhosis and Rheumathoid Arthritis are associated with peptic ulcers.
- Clinical Presentation and Diagnosis:
    o Peptic ulcers may occur at any age but more common between 12-18 years. Boys are affected more than the girls.
    o Young children present with vomiting and upper gastrointestinal bleeding while older children present with epigastric pain and occult gastrointestinal bleeding. The pain is relieved by food or anti acids and recurring 2 hours after eating. It typically wakes the child from sleep.
    o H. Pylori is diagnosed by:

- - -
            - Serology tests which shows previous exposure to this gram-ve organism.
            - Urea breath test for urease which is + ve in about 90% of cases.
            - Histology by testing gastric tissue for urease activity.
            - Culture and PCR testing.
        - Barium meal study may show an ulcer crater. 25% of cases could be missed by this test.
        - Upper intestinal endoscopy is the most accurate diagnostic test for peptic ulcer.
- Treatment is directed to:
    - Reduce gastric activity by:
        - Antiacids but they are poorly tolerated and their action is short lived.
        - H2 receptor antagonists such as Cimetidine (5mg/kg/dose, 4 doses/day) or Ranitidine (2.5mg/kg/dose every 12 hours) produce healing in 6 weeks and provide sustained relief for 6-12 months.
        - Proton pump inhibitors (Omeprazole and Iansoprazole) inhibit gastric acid secretion by the parietal cells.
    - Eradication of H. Pylori infection, if present. This is done by the combination of Clarithromycin, Metronidazole and Bismuth salts for 7-14 days.
    - Avoid food that causes pain, caffeine, Aspirin and NSAIDS.
    - Surgical vagotomy with pyloroplasty is only indicated in perforated uncontrolled bleeding, intractable pain or obstruction.

Intussusception

- Intussusception is invagination of one segment of the bowel into another. The ileocolic form is the most frequent, then ileoileal and colocolic.
- It is the most frequent cause of intestinal obstruction in the first 2 years life. Male to female is 3:1.

- In the majority of cases the causes is unknown, but it is thought that viral infections with lymphoid hyperplasia of Peyer patches forming the lead point of the proximal in intussusceptions segment may be reason.
- In older children the predisposing factors include: Polyps, Meckel's diverticulum, Lymphomas, Lypoms, Parasites and Henoch-Schonlein Purpura. Bulk of stool in the terminal ileum seen in Cystic Fibrosis and Coeliac disease might lead to intussusception.
- Clinical presentation is typically as follows:
    o Intermittent severe colicky abdominal pain with screaming and drowning up of the knees occurring in otherwise healthy infant aged 3-12 months.
    o Between the attacks he appears comfortable.
    o Vomiting occurring soon after that in most cases. It is nonbilious initially but becomes bilious as the obstruction worsens.
    o Diarrhea occurs and in 50% of cases patients might later pass current jelly stools with mixed blood and mucus.
    o Lethargy and low grade fever supervene.
    o A Sausage-shape mass may be palpable in the upper mid abdomen,
    o Abdominal X-rays reveal a distended small bowel obstruction. A mass or the actual intussusception may also be seen.
    o Barium enema is both diagnostic and therapeutic. It may reduce a simple intussusception in 75% of the case. It should not be performed if peritonitis due to perforation is suspected.
    o Air insufflation of the colon under fluoroscopic guidance is a safer alternative.
    o Surgical reduction should be performed if there is perforation or if the medical reduction is unsuccessful or in very ill patients.
    o In few cases intussusception recurs within 24hrs after medical reduction. This is seen much less after surgical reduction. Multiple intussusception at the same have been reported.

Acute Appendicitis

- This is a common cause of acute abdominal pain and the most common indication for emergency abdominal surgery in childhood.
- Appendicitis should be considered in all ages but more commonly between 4-16 years of age.
- Predisposing Factors include:
    o Obstruction of the appendix by fecaliths (in 25% of the cases).
    o Obstruction by lymphatic hyperplasia from a non specific infection.
    o Obstruction by parasites
    o Meconium ileus equivalent
    o Drugs e.g. Vincristine
- Clinical Presentation is typical in only about 50% of the cases. It includes:
    o Vague central abdominal pain is the earliest symptom
    o Fever which is usually low grade. High fever suggests perforation.
    o Anorexia, nausea and vomiting
    o The pain remains constant but with in 24 - 48hrs shifts to the right iliac fossa as the local parietal peritoneal inflammation develops. This is Mc Burney point.
    o Diarrhea or sometimes constipation may be present.
    o Physical examination which should be repeated till a final diagnosis settled, will show tenderness and rebound tenderness in the right iliac fossa. The child will be lying very still, usually on one side with or without knees flexed. Movement or cough worsens the pain. Deep palpation of the left iliac fossa may cause pain in the right iliac fossa. This is Rovsing's sign.
    o Other causes of abdominal pain like pneumonia should be ruled out by careful examination.
- A typical clinical picture is common. This might lead to delay in the diagnosis of appendicitis with development of perforation. These include:
    o Watery diarrhea which might result in diagnosing gastroenteritis

- o Generalized abdominal pain with tenderness around the umbilicus and high fever which might lead to the diagnosis of mesenteric adenitis.
- o Intermittent abdominal pain
- o Retrocecal appendix gives less peritoneal irritation. If the inflamed appendix is on the psoas muscles, the patient will lie in his RT hip flexed to relief the pain. This is psoas sign.
- o Pelvic appendix makes rectal examination an essential examination that should always be done in all cases. It will reveal localized tenderness and a mass.
- o Whenever in doubt, an abdominal ultrasound examination should be done because of it high sensitivity and specificity. Accumulation of fluid in the lumen of an enlarged and incompressible appendix surrounded by fluid is a major finding in the case of non perforated appendix. This is donut or target sign.
- o CT scan of the abdomen may be diagnostic in difficult cases.
- o Surgical condition should be seaked early to exclude appendicitis in any child with abdominal complaints which do not settle quickly. The risk of perforation greatly increases with time.
- Differential diagnosis includes: gastroenteritis, urinary track infection, mesenteric adenitis, pneumonia, constipation, intussusception, Meckel's diverticulum, Henoch-Schonlein purpura and hepatitis.
- Treatment is appendectomy of the acutely inflamed appendix. A single pre-operative dose of antibiotics like ceftriaxone, cefitaxime reduces the incidence of post operative wound infection. For patients gangrenous or perforated appendix, a broad spectrum antibiotics effective against anaerobic and gram-ve enteric organisms are given.

Peritonitis

- It could be primary or secondary.

- Primary bacteria peritonitis is very rare. It occurs in the following patients:
    - o Patients with splenic dysfunction or who had splenectomy.
    - o Patients with ascites due to Nephrotic syndrome, liver disease, Kwashiorkor.
    - o Patients with pyelonephritis or pneumonia.
- Primary peritonitis is caused by pneumococci, Group A B-haemolytic streptococci and E. coli, TB
- Secondary peritonitis occurs in the following conditions:
    - o Perforated or ruptured bowel which complicates conditions like appendicitis.
    - o In patients with Necrotizing enterocolitis
    - o Penetrating abdominal trauma
    - o Patients on peritoneal dialysis.
- Secondary peritonitis is caused by organism like Staphylococcus epidermidis, Bacteroids, Candida.
- Clinical presentation of peritonitis include:
    - o Severe abdominal pain
    - o Fever usually above 39°
    - o Vomiting with anorexia
    - o Diarrhea is a common early symptom in primary peritonitis but later become constipated.
    - o The abdomen is distended, tender to touch and rigid.
- Investigation will show very high WBC and blood culture positive in primary peritonitis.
- Paracentesis is the diagnostic test if the fluid shows:
    - o Polymorph nucleated leukocytes more than 500 cells/micro
    - o Gram stain reveals the organism.
    - o Exudative fluid
- Abdominal ultrasound will confirm the diagnosis.
- Treatment is by giving appropriate antibiotics together with supportive therapy. Underlying cause of secondary peritonitis should be treated surgically as soon as possible.

Achalasia of the Oesophagus

- This is failure of relaxation of the lower esophageal sphincter during swallowing. There is abnormal peristalsis in the esophageal body. It could be of familial (Allgrove Syndrome) or acquired aetiology or idiopathic.
- Clinical presentation: The classical picture is seen after the age of 5 years as:
    o Dysphagia with food sticking on the upper chest which is relieved by vomiting or repeated forceful swallowing.
    o Chronic cough and wheezing resembling asthma.
    o Recurrent aspiration pneumonitis.
- In a well established case, barium swallow will show a dilated upper oesophagus with a narrow short distal part.
- Esophageal manometry may show abnormal or absent peristalsis and high resting pressure in the lower esophagus.
- Treatment is by:
    o Dilation of the lower esophageal sphincter by balloon.
    o Heller myotomy which is surgical splitting of the lower esophageal sphincter muscle.

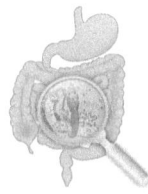

INFLAMMATORY BOWEL DISEASE

- These mainly include Crohn's disease, ulcerative colitis and few indeterminate colitis.
- The etiology of the conditions is unknown but most likely it is an abnormal genetic predisposition to an immunologic or inflammatory response to an environmental antigenic factor. This is probably and infection of a sort.
- Crohn's disease is twice as common as ulcerative colitis in the UK and it may involve any part of the entire gastrointestinal tract from mouth to the anal canal. Ulcerative colitis involves only the colon rectum (95% of cases) and its incidence is more in the U.S.A than Crohn's disease.
- They cause bowel inflammation with symptoms of diarrhea, abdominal pain, fever and passing blood. They differ in other features.
- Both may have extra intestinal manifestations that could be the predominate presenting symptoms for both, making the right diagnosis difficult. These include:
    - Arthritis/ Arthralgia
    - Stomatitis
    - Uveitis/ conjunctivitis/ episcleritis
    - Erythema Nodosum
    - Renal stones
    - Chronic active hepatitis
    - Sclerosing cholangitis which is seen only in 4% of ulcerate colitis patient.

Crohn's Disease

- Because Crohn's disease may involve any part of the G.I. tract its symptoms may be mistaken for any other diseases.
- Anorexia and weight loss is seen in most patients. This malnutrition is not only caused by anorexia but also by malabsorption caused by diarrhea, protein-losing enteropathy and disaccharidase deficiency
- 10-15% of cases presented in childhood, usually during teenage.
- The common presenting symptoms are diarrhea, abdominal pain, and weight loss. Abdominal masses (granulomas) are commonly felt.
- The acute and chronic inflammation in trans mural (full thickness) in a discontinuous pattern.
- Perianal manifestations like skin tags, fissures, fistulas and abscess are common in Crohn's disease. Intestinal obstruction is also common but perforation and haemorrhage are rare.
- The risk of colon cancer is rare in Crohn's disease.
- Diagnosis: The above clinical picture strongly suggests the diagnosis. Test done:
    o Blood tests will show leukocytosis, high ESR, positive CRP, low serum protein and anaemia.
    o Barium study may show small bowel lesions especially in the ilium, large bowel disease with skipped areas segmental of narrowing the so called string sign.
    o Gastroscopy and colonoscopy with biopsy of the affected area will confirm pathology.
- Treatments are discussed with the treatment ulcerative colitis as they are similar in many ways.

Ulcerative Colitis

- The inflammatory manifestation of ulcerative colitis is limited to the colon and rectal mucosa. It is not transmural as in Crohn disease but only a supperficial acute inflammation of the mucosa with microscopic crypt abscess. A backwash ileitis s often seen.
- It is more common in females than male.

- The disease could be mild, moderate or severe, but all have blood in stool and most present with abdominal pain, with tenesmous in three quarters of the patients.
- Mild cases are those with less than four stools per day, with no fever, no anemia and no hypoalbunemia. It mimics irritable bowel syndrome.
- Severe cases are those with more than 10 stools per day, with severe anemia, high fever, severe bleeding and leukocytosis.
- The disease can present predominantly with extra intestinal manifestation.
- Toxic mega colon is a serious complocation seen in 5% of cases of ulcerative colitis. Carcinoma of the colon may occur in long standing cases, so routine cancer screening is recommended in patients with 10 years pancolitis manifestation.
- Barium enema with a double contrast will show diffuse superficial colitis with loss of normal haustrations in the colon (the so called lead-pipe appearance) Pseudopolyps are late findings.
- Endoscopy and biopsy which shows the classical histological features is the dignostic procedure of choice.
- The medical treatment of ulcerative colitis and Crohn's disease is similar and includes anti-inflammatory therapy, antibiotics medication and dietary modifications.
    - o The most widely used treatment in pediatric practice is enteral nutrition used exclusively for 4-8 weeks followed by gradual reintroduction of diet which is high in protein, high in carbohydrates with normal amount of fat. Vitamins and iron supplements should be given. Enteral administration of elemental liquid diet is better started first. Relapses may occur with normal diet.
    - o Sulfasalazine given orally is effective in mild cases of ulcerative colitis and in Crohn disease of the colon. The drug prevents relapse of ulcerative colitiis once remission is induced. It is not absorbed in the small intestine and it inhibits folic acid absorption. It also causes skin rash, pancreatitis, hemolytic aplastic anemia, rarely.
    - o Conticosteroids as oral predmisolone 1-2mg/kg/day is given with sulfasalazine to moderate cases.

- o Severe cases are treated with I.V. steroids together with enteral nutrition and careful monitoring of electrolytes inbalance and acid base adjustments. Hydrocortisone enemas are also used. Prednisolone is the most effective drug for Crohn's disease of the small intestine.
- o Azathioprine 1-2mg/kg/day and 6 mercaptopurine are used in cases of corticosteroid dependence or resistance. Methotrexate can be used when those drugs fail. These drugs may cause myelo suppression, so regular blood counts are required.
- o Metronidazole is an effective drug in cases of Crohn's disease with perianal manifestations.
- o Surgical treatment is eventically needed in 70% of patients with Crohn's disease and about 25% of patients with ulcertative colitis for failed medical treatment. Surgery is colectomy with ileotomy in some. Ileoanal ansstomosis is performed.
- Other causes of colitis should always be excluded. These include:
  - o Inefective causes of colitis caused by:
    - Shigella
    - Salmonela
    - Yersinia
    - Cambylobacter
    - Entamoeba hystolitica causing amoebiasis.
    - Invasive E.coli and toxin producing E.coli.
    - Clostridium difficile causing pseudomembranous colitis.
    - CMV causing colitis.
    - Tuberculosis
  - o Non-infective colitis
    - Behcet's disease
    - Food allergy colitis
    - Enterobius vermiculosis
    - Undetermined colitis

Gastrointestinal bleeding

- Gastrointestinal bleeding may present as hematemesis, or malaenia or passing fresh blood per rectum. It is an alarming symptoms that needs careful history to identify the bleeding source. Firstly, it is important to confirm that it is real blood and it is coming from the gastrointestinal track of the patient.
- Physical examination to assess the patient's condition is very important to evaluate how much blood has been lost and if the patient is still bleeding.

Haematemesis

- This is vomiting of bright red blood or coffee ground material. If there is no associated blood in the stool, this implies that the site of the bleeding is proximal to the ligament of Treitz.
  The causes of hematemesis include:
    o Swallowed maternal blood in a neonate. Apt test will differentiate between fetal and maternal blood.
    o Swallowed blood after epistaxis or bleeding in oropharynx.
    o Hemorragic disease of new born.
    o Gastroesophageal reflux with oesophagitis/Hiatus Hernia.
    o Oesophageal varices
    o Gastritis due to irritation by ingestion of corrosive drugs like Aspirin and NSAID.
    o Peptic ulcer
    o Mallony-Weiss syndrome with excessive vomiting causing mucosal tear.
    o Severe infections like haemorrhagic fever, rarely malaria.
    o Blood diseases e.g. Thrombocytopenia, DIC, Leukaemia, Aplastic Anemia.
    o Protein milk allergy may rarely cause haematemesis
    o Scurvy
    o Tumours of the G-I tract.
    o Rendu-Osler-Weber Syndrome
    o Munchausen Syndrome by Proxy when blood is placed in the vomitus.

Malaenia and passing fresh blood per rectum

- Malaenia is the passage of black stools due to the presence of blood altered by intestinal juices, so it is due to upper gastrointestinal bleeding, proximal to the ileocecal valve.
- Haematochezia is the passage of frank gross blood in the stool and indicates lower gastrointestinal tract bleeding, most frequentky colonic.
- Causes of Malaenia and Haematochezia include:
    o Anal fissure in all age groups
    o Infectious diarrhoea
    o Nectrotizing Enterocolitis
    o Volvulus
    o Hirschsprung disease
    o Meckel Diverticulum
    o Intussusception
    o Gastrointestinal duplication/ Malrotation of the gut.
    o Gastritis/ Peptic ulcer
    o Swallowed blood
    o Protein milk allergy
    o Crohn's Disease
    o Ulcerative colitis
    o Juvenile polyps/ familial polyposis/ Peutz- Jeghers Syndrome
    o Henosh- Schonlein Purpura
    o Blood diseases as in haematemesis
    o Diverticulitis
    o Severe Congential heart disease/ Acute intestinal ischaemia
    o Drugs

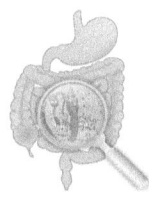

VOMITING

- It is a very common symptom in pediatric medicine. It may cause by a number of problems in many organ system of the body.
- It is defined as the forceful coordinated act of expelling abdominal contents through the mouth.
- To be able to reach to the underlying cause of vomiting should focus on the following clinical features:
    o The age of the patient whether aneonate, infant, yough or old child. Intestinal obstruction should be considered in a neonate who is vomiting. One should look for another symptoms and signs of obstruction in the young patients.
    o Type of the vomitus gastrict contents vomiting is characteristic of pyloric stenosis. It is also seen in infections like UTI an otitis media as well as inpeptic disease, CNS problems and Renal disorder. Bile stained vomiting may be due to small intestinal obstruction. Bloody vomitus may be due to bleeding peptic ulcer, oesophageal varic bleeding disorder or some other causes.
    o Other associated symptoms and signs. Abdominal sysmptoms like diarrhea may indicate the gastroenterities while extra abdominal symptoms like headaches and toxic look may be due to meningitis.
    o Detailed history and careful physical examination followed by specific investigations is the key to the diagnosis.

Causes of Vomiting

- Excessive Regurgitation
- Gastroesophageal Reflux
- Hiatus hernia/ Diaphragmatic hernia
- Achalasia
- Oesophageal Atresia and Stenosis
- Gastrointestinal obstruction anomalies (all congenital causes)
- Necrotizing enterocolitis in prematures
- Gastroenteritis
- Inborn errors of metabolism (Urea cycle, Amino acids, Organic aciduria)
- Congenital adrenal hyperplasia
- Intussusception
- Milk allergy and intollerance
- Food allergy and Coeliac disease
- Peptic disease with or without ulcers
- Appendicitis
- Hepatitis
- Pancreatitis
- Ascaris
- Septicanemia
- Whooping cough
- Urunary Track Infections
- Obstructive Uropathy
- Uremia
- Meningitis
- Kernicterus
- Subdural haematoma
- Hydrocephalus
- Cerebral oedema
- Intracranial space occupying lesion
- Lead encephalopathy
- Drug toxicity e.g. Theophyline, Aspirin
- Motion sickness
- Migraine in an old child
- Diabetic Ketoacidosis
- Reye's Syndrome

- Psychogenic
- Coeliac crises can be seen in very ill patients as follows:
    o Severe diarrhoea
    o Profound malnutrition
    o Abdominal distension
    o Peripheral oedema
    o Hypokalaemia
    o Acidosis
    o Dehydration
    o Shock
- Steroids are given to the patient in Coeliac crises as well as correcting the dehydration and the electrolyte imbalance.
- Malignant lymphoma of the small bowel and other gastrointestinal malignancies may occur in long standing cases if the diet is not adhered to.

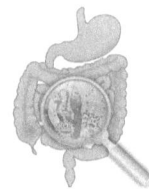

DIARRHOEAL DISEASES

- More than 90% of the fluid (water and electrolyte) entering the small intestine is absorbed by the villi. The rest goes to the large bowel where further absorption occurs leaving only about 100-200 mls of water which is excreted in stools per day.
- The crypts of the bowel epithelium secrete fluid into the lumen. Diarrhea will result if there is reduced absorption by the villi or increased secretion by the crypts, or both.
- Diarrhea is defined as a change in bowel habit for an individual child to an increase in the stool water content. It is not a disease but a symptom to a disease.
- Young infants may have 3-10 stools per day depending on the method of feeding as breast fed have more frequent stools. Old infants and toddlers usually have 1-2 stools per day.
- Worldwide, diarrhea remain one of the most common illnesses among children in developing countries there are about 1.5 billion episodes of diarrhea and 4 million associated deaths among children each year. These WHO statistics translate to an average of 3.3eposide of diarrhea per year for each child less than year 5 years of age.

Causes of diarrhoea

1. **Infections**
    A) Gastrointestinal (Enteral)
    - Viruses: Rotavirus, Norwalk virus, Enteroviruses, astroviruses

- Bacterial: salmonella, shigella, yersinia, Campylobacter, pathogenic, Escherichia coli, Aeromonas Hydrophilia, Vibrio spp., Clostridium difficile, Tuberculosis
- Parasites: Giardia lamblia, Entamoeba histolytica.

B) Non-gastrointestinal (Parenteral)
- Upper respiration tract infection may present with diarrhoea
- Systemic infections may cause diarrhoea e.g. UTI, pneumonia, Otitis media

2. Dietary Disturbances

- Food allergy
- Over feeding
- Starvation

3. Surgical condition

- Intussusception
- Appendicitis
- Hirschsprung's disease
- Partial obstruction
- Blind loop syndrome

4. Inflammatory bowel Disease

- Ulcerative colitis
- Crohn's disease

5. Malabsorption

- Cystic fibrosis
- Coeliac disease
- Disaccharides deficiency
- Acrodermatitis Enteropathica
- Intestinal lymphangiectasia

6. Psychogenic disturbances (imitable bowel syndrome)

7. **Systemic diseases**

    - Endocrine diseases e.g. hyperthyroidism, hypoparathyroidism, congenital adrenal hyperplasia.
    - Immune deficiency

8. **Miscellaneous**

    - Antibiotic associated diarrhea
    - Secondary lactase deficiency
    - Neonatal drug withdrawal
    - Haemolytic Uraemic syndrome

    - The most common causes of diarrhea are the infective gastroenteritis due to viruses, followed by dietary disturbances, irritable bowel syndrome, the antibiotic associated diarrhoea and the diarrhoea secondary to lactose intolerance.
    - The most serious causes of diarrhoea are the intussusception, Hirschsprung disease, toxic mega colon due to inflammatrory bowel disease, haemolytic uraemic syndrome, neonatal salmonella infection and the pseudomembranous colitis.
    - Although gastroenteritis is the commonest cause of diarrhoea, the following features may indicate a diagnosis other than acute gastroenteritis:
        - Severe abdominal pain with tenderness/guarding and/ or bilious vomiting is most likely due to surgical causes.
        - Pallor, jaundice, oliguria, bloody stools may indicate haemolytic uraemic syndrome.
        - Child is generally unwell with systemic manifestations out of proportion to the level of dehydration, most likely this is due to a systemic infection or surgical cause or congenital adrenal hyperplasia.
    - Diagnosing the cause of diarrhoea depends on taking detailed history and performing physical examination.
    - The following are important features in the history:
    Duration of the diarrhea is the important diagnostic to different between acute diarrhea (lasting less than 2 weeks) and chronic diarrhea. Acute diarrhea is mainly due to infective causes and

less commonly to surgical causes. Chronic diarrhea may be due to inflammatory bowel diseases, malabsorption, irritable bowel syndrome, dietary disturbances and systemic diseases.
- History of fever in acute diarrhea indicates an infective cause.
- Temperature more than 39.5c suggests bacterial enteritis.
- Bloody diarrhea suggests bacterial gastro enteritis which is the commonest cause of bloody direction. Occasionally viral gastro enteritis may cause bloody diarrhea.
- Inflammatory bowel disease may cause bloody diarrhea, also pseudo membranous colitis.

– Other points in history that helps in the diagnosis and management of diarrhea
Include:
- Frequency of diarrhea, consistency and volume of stools
- Associated vomiting, its frequency and colour of vomitus.
- Associated abdominal pain and the site of the pain.
- Urinary symptoms and the amount and colour of urine.
- Feeding history, type of feeding (breast or bottle), amount of feeds, how formula feeds are constituted, amount of fluids taken during the illness
- Ask about weight loss and if it is recent or over a larger period of time
- Family history of similar diarrhoea and type of food taken
- Any recent travel
- Past medical history of similar attacks of diarrhoea.
- History of food allergy or any other allergic manifestations
- Any antibiotics taken prior to the diarrhea attack
- History of associated acute illness e.g. tonsillitis, otitis media, pneumonia, convulsion
- History of systemic diseases e.g. thyroid disease

Clinical examination:
- Observe level of consciousness and behavior
- Assess the degree of dehydration
- Look for signs of shock (weak rapid pulse, capillary refill, cold extremities, hypotension)
- Look for pallor, presence of purpura and any other rash
- Check temp. and weight of the child

- Look for hair changes to exclude malnutrition and accrodermatitis enteropathica.
- ENT examination for evidence of infection.
- Neck examination for lymphadenopathy and thyroid enlargement.
- Chest examination for evidence of pneumonia.
- Heart examination for abnormal heart beats and rate.
- Examination for abnormal masses, tenderness and sign of obstruction. Rectal examination for masses and to obtain stools for examination or take rectal swab for c/s.
- CNS examination to exclude serious infections and to look for signs of electrolyte disturbances, checking tone, power and reflexes.
- Examine lower extremities for muscle wasting which is seen in malabsorption syndrome.

- **Investigations:**
    - Stool examination for:
        - Microscopic examination for cells, ova, cysts and parasites.
        - Culture of fresh stools for bacteria.
        - Elisa test for Rota virus.
        - Stools pH and reducing substances. If pH is <6 then CHO malabsorption may present. Colour, consistency, odour, mucous, blood and pus cells.
        - Stools for occult blood.
    - Urinalysis and culture.
    - Blood for Hb (anemia may be seen in coeliac disease), WBC, platelets and ESR.
    - Serum electrolytes, blood pH and bicarbonate.
    - Blood culture.
    - Blood for area and creatinine.

[I] ACUTE DIARRHOEA

(1) Viral gastro enteritis

- Viral gastro enteritis is a common illness that occurs in both endemic and epidemic forms worldwide. It accounts for 80% of acute diarrhea in developed countries.
- Viral intestinal infection decreases the absorptive surface of the small bowel. This type of lesion takes about 3-7 days to heal.
- The clinical presentation of viral gastro enteritis is as follows:
    - Incubation period is very short, 1-2days
    - Vomiting is usually the first symptoms in about 80%of patients
    - Low grade fever then develops
    - Diarrhea which is profuse and watery follows within 24 hours and may last for about a weak. The stool dose not contain blood or white cells.
    - Infants become dehydrated rapidly
    - Metabolic acidosis may develop due to bicarbonate loss in the stools.
- There are 4 types of viruses that are known to cause human gastro enteritis. These are Rota virus, Enteric Adeno virus, Calicivirus including Norwalk virus and Astrovirus.

A) Rota Virus

- Human Rota virus was first detected in 1973 by electron microscopy in duodenal biopsy samples of children with acute gastroenteritis by Bishop. Because of the circular outline of the outer surface of the virus resembles a double-rimed wheel, it is called Rota which in Latin means wheel.
- Rota virus is the most common viral infection to cause gastroenteritis in infants. It accounts for about 40% of diarrhoea-related hospitalization among children aged <5 years, occurring mainly during winter. It is the major cause of death among children in many developing countries.
- The virus is transmitted mainly by the faecal oral route. Also waterborne transmission may occur in public swimming pools.

It may rarely spread by infected respiratory droplets coughed or sneezed in air. Incubation period is 1-3 days.
- The virus invades the intestinal mucosal cell and produce enterotoxins which cause villous damage. Large quantities of virus are shed in faeses from just prior to onset of symptoms until about 10 days after onset of symptoms.
- Infants present with the triad of repeated vomiting, fever and profuse diarrhoea which is watery, foul smelling and may last for 8 days. Occasionally the stool contains mucous and blood. Dehydration develops rapidly and may lead to death. Hypernatremia may develop, the stool sodium is usually <40meq/l. many children have concomitant rhinorrhea.
- Diagnosis of Rota virus may be made by rapid antigen detection of the virus in stools using Enzyme immunoassay (ELISA) or Latex agglutination test for fast detection.
- Electron microscopy for detection of the virus in the stool is used in research labs. Reverse transcription-polymerase chain reaction (RT-PCR) can detect all types of Rota virus, but it is not used clinically.
- Serotype GIP (8) is the most common serotype worldwide causing the infection and accounting for > two thirds of Rota virus infection.
- The initial infection is most likely severe with subsequent infections more commonly mild or asymptomatic. Subsequent infections are almost always of a different serotype.
- At risk group to develop infection includes children in day care centres and their parents/caretakers, children in hospitals and their parents, and children with immune deficiency syndromes.
- Prevention of Rota virus:
  1) Apart from improved hygiene and use of clean water, breast feeding helps to reduce the incidence of Rota virus infection.
  2) Vaccination against Rota virus is now used successfully. There are two vaccines, Rota Teq vaccine (by Merk) with 3 doses at ages 2month, 4month and 6month, and Rotarix vaccine (by Glaxo Smith Kline Co) with 2 doses before the age of 6 month. Intussusception does not occur with these vaccines.

B) Enteric Adenoviruses

- This is the second most common cause of viral gastroenteritis in infants and children worldwide. It causes symptoms similar to Rota virus but they are generally less severe. It occurs in children younger than 2 years of age.
- Diarrhoea is the most prominent symptom and can last from 4days to 3weeks. Blood and mucous are not seen in the stools. Dehydration is mild and death is rare. In immunocompromised patients the infection is associated with increased mortality and prolonged hospitalization.
- Members of the household may be infected at the same time. The virus is transmitted by faecal-oral route. The infection occurs all year round but increases in summer.
- Diagnosis is by detection of antigen in stools using commercially available kits PCR and electron microscopy are used in research labs.

C) Calciviruses and calci-like virus including Norwalk virus

- Caliciviruses have a worldwide distribution and are a common cause of water and food borne outbreaks of acute non bacterial gastro enteritis. The outbreaks tend to occur in closed population and have a high attack rate.
- Caliciviruses cause illness more frequently among infants and children while Norwalk viruses, which are regarded as a form of caliciviruses, cause illness among older children and adults.
- Norwalk virus, now named Norovirus, was the first gastro enteritis virus discovered. It was identified first in 1972 when an outbreak of gastroenteritis occurred in a school in Norwalk city in USA.
- Norwalk virus typically present with nausea and vomiting "winter vomiting"
  Diarrhoea and abdominal pain occur in most cases. Fever and chills may be present. The incubation period is 1-3 days and the illness usually last longer than 4 days
- Diagnosis can be made by identification of Norwalk virus antigen in stools.

Tests like enzyme immunoassay (EIA) that use antibodies (e.g. RIDASCREEN test) are recently used. Specific diagnosis is made by polymerase chain reaction (PCR) assay. The virus can be identified by electron microscopy.

D) Astroviruses

- Astroviruses were first described in 1975. They typically affect children less than 7 years of age. The infection is seen mainly during winter.
- The infection is transmitted by contact among children and by faecal oral route. Outbreaks were reported due to contaminated water and shellfish
- The incubation period is 24-36 hours with the illness lasting 1-4 days. The symptoms of vomiting, diarrhoea and fever are milder than the Rota virus infection. Asymptomatic infections also occur.
- Diagnosis can be made by ELISA, PCR, immuno fluorescence and Reverse Transcription-Polymerase Chain (RT-PCR). The virus is identified by electron microscope.

(2) Bacterial Gastroenteritis

- Bacterial G-E accounts for 10-15% of diagnosed gastro enteritis in children in developed countries. The term dysentery refers to abdominal cramps, tenesmus and blood and pus in stools. Bacteria is the commonest cause of bloody diarrhoea
- The commonest bacteria that cause diarrhoea are: A) Salmonella, B) Shigella, C) Campylobacter, D) Pathogenic E.Coli, E) Yersinia.
- Stools general examination and culture are the diagnostic methods for bacteria G-E. A thin smear of fresh stool is placed on a slide and air-dried. Methylene blue is poured on the sample for 5 seconds than gently rinsed with tap water and air- dried again. The sample is examined under high-power field microscope to detect the neutrophils (pus cells). RBC are seen in the microscopic examination.

  The culture of the stool will confirm the presence and type of bacteria.

- Bacteria causes diarrhoea by a number of mechanisms:
1-Bacteria enter the gastro intestinal tract where it causes diarrhoea by one of the following ways:
    - Bacteria invade the mucosa of the intestinal tract, grow and multiply within the mucosal cells, as in salmonella, shigella and some E.coli infection.
    - Bacteria secret cytotoxins that damage the intestinal cells causing its dysfunction and leading to profuse diarrhoea, as in enterohaemmorrhic E.coli, Shigella and Clostridium difficile

Bacteria secrete enterotoxins which cause altered cell salt and water balance, without damaging the structure of the cells, by leading to the
    - inhibition of absorption of water and salt by the villi, as seen in V.Chlolrae and enterotoxic E.coli
    - Bacteria adhere to the cell membrane of the mucosa of both small and large intestine and secrete enterotoxins that cause flattening of the microvilli, as seen in some E.coli infection.

2-Bacteria secrete preformed exotoxins that are then ingested by the host and attack the intestinal mucosa causing diarrhoea within hours, as in staph. food poisoning and botulism.

A) Salmonella G.E (Non-typhi salmonella)

- Salmonella infection is caused by contaminated food products like milk, egg and poultry or transmitted through contact with infected animals like chicken.
- The incubation period is 8-48 hours. Symptoms are abdominal pain, nausea, watery diarrhoea, which may be bloody, and fever. There will mild leukocytosis and the stool examination will show polymophs neutrophils of moderate degree. Stool culture will be diagnostic

B) Shigella G-E

- Transmitted by faecal oral route through foods like salad, row vegetable, tuna meat, shrimps, milk and dairy products.

- There are 4 types of Shigella: S. sonnei which is the commonest type in developed countries, S. flexneri which is the commonest in the developing world, S.dysenteriae which causes the most severe form of the disease including HUS, and S. boydii.
- Shigella is transmitted by faecal-oral route and is passed easily from person to person as only 10 organisms can cause the infection. The incubation period is 12-48 hours.
- Shigella may cause an asymptomatic disease, mild gastroenteritis or bacillary dysentery.
    - Mild disease is the commonest form. Children present with frequently watery diarrhoea but few constitutional symptoms. The temperature is usually normal but some may have low grade fever.
    - Bacillary dysentery: children present with sudden onset of fever and abdominal pain. Diarrhoea then develops shortly afterwards, as frequent motions which usually contains mucus and blood. Tenesmus is common. Colitis may develop. 10-30% of children may develop seizures.
    - Complications of Shigella infection include dehydration, hyponatraemia, hypoglycaemia, encephalopathy and seizures, haemolytic uraemic syndrome (HUS), intestinal perforation, pneumonia and malnutrition. These lead to death in 1/4 of the children in developing countries.
- Diagnosis in shigella: stool smear will show polymorphonuclear leucocytes arranged in sheets. Stool culture are usually positive but may be negative in some patients. blood shows increased WBC with marked shift to the left. Leukemoid reaction may be seen in 10% of the cases with WBC > 50,000.
- Serological tests are used to identify different species. An enzyme immunoassay is used to detected S dysentiae type1. PCR assay is used in specialized labs.

C) Campylabacter G.E

- Campylobacter infection is transmitted by person to person contact and by contaminated water and food. The bacteria invades the mucosa of the jejunum, ileum and colon causing entero colitis. The incubation period is 1-7 days

- The infection is characterized by the sudden onset of fever, which may reach 40C in older children, and abdominal pain. The diarrhoea follows soon as watery stools which usually contain blood. Vomiting is uncommon. The disease lasts for 2-7 days.
- In tropical countries asymptotic stool carriage is common. Relapse of the disease occurs in up to 1/4 of the patients.
- Stool smear will show polymorph leukocytes and RBC. Blood shows leukocytosis of mild degree. Stool culture will isolate the bacteria but it needs special preparations and special media. Dark field or phase-contrast microscopy of faecal specimens for characteristic darting motility within 2hrs of passing stools can be used.
- A gram stain of stools samples for characteristic curved rods is specific with a sensitivity of 50-75%.

D) E. coli

- E.coli may cause diarrhoea of varying types and severity by several distinct mechanisms:
    - i) EPEC (Entropathogenic E. coli). This is the classic E.coli which cause a characteristic histologic injury in the small bowel, adherence and effacement. It is responsible for many of the epidemics of diarrhoea in nurseries for neonates and in day care centres.
    - ii) ETEC (Entrotoxigenic E.coli) This usually produces enterotoxins causing mild, self limiting illness without significant fever or systemic toxicity. It plays a major role in traveler's diarrhoea. In newborns and infants it may cause severe diarrhoea.
    - iii) EIEC (Enteroinvasive E.coli) This usually invades the colonic mucosa causing widespread mucosal damage with acute inflammation. It causes Shigela-like illness with fever, systemic symptoms, bloody diarrhoea and leulcocytosis.
    - iv) EHEC (Enterohaemorrhagic E.coli) this causes haemorrhagic colitis, especially E. coli 0157:H7 strain. Diarrhoea is initially watery then become bloody. Abdominal pain and cramps occur but no fever. HUS occurs within days in 2-5% of children.

E) Yersina G-E

- Infants and young children characteristically have diarrhoea while old children usually have acute lesions of the terminal ileum or acute mesenteric adenitis resembling appendicitis.
- The onset of diarrhoea is sudden with frequent watery stools that may contain blood. There is severe abdominal pain but vomiting is uncommon. Fever may develop. Arthritis and skin rash occur in 5 to 10% of patients. The disease is self-limited lasting 3days to 3 weeks.
- The WBC is usually normal. The stool smear shows polymorph nuclear leulcocytes.

Features suggestive of bacterial rather than viral gaster enteritis

- The followings are features suggestive of bacterial rather than viral gastro- enteritis:

    1-More than 10 stools per day or diarrhea lasting for more than 4 days
    2-Blood in stool
    3-Fever greater than 39.5C
    4-Clinical toxicity
    5-Polymorphonuclear leucocytes in the stools

Management of bacterial gastro ententis

A) Salmonella G-E (Non-typhi)

- Salmonella gastro enteritis is usually a self limiting condition. Antibiotics should not be given in such cases. Infants less than 6 months and children with sickle cell disease may develop severe infections like septicaemia, meningitis and osteomyelitis.
- Children with Salmonella G.E that need hospitalization:
    - Dehydrated children
    - Evidence of focal infection or septicaemia
    - Infants less than 3 months of age

- Fever greater than 38.5c in an infant less than 12 month of age
- Sickle cell anaemia patients
- If septicaemia is suspected (or osteomyelitis) adequate hydration is given together with I.V. Ampicillin 200mg/kg/day or ceftriaxone 100mg/kg/day or ciprofloxacin is given until sensitivity is available.

B) Shigellosis

- Mild cases recover without antibiotics treatment. An adequate hydration with ORS should be given. Anti diarrheal drugs like Lomotil (diphenoxylate + atropine) should not be given because of the risk of prolongation of the disease.
- Severe cases with bacillary dysentery are treated with antibiotics. Although most cases can be handled on an out patient basis, the following will require hospitalization:
    - Patients under the age of 6 month. Neonates get infected from asymptomatic mothers.
    - Dehydrated patients.
    - Patients who show evidence of bacteraemia or other complications of the disease.
    - Malnourished children and immuno suppressed patients.
- The antibiotics that are effective against Shigella include: Trimethoprim/sulfamethoxazole (Septrin), Ampicillin, Ceftriaxone, Ciprofloxacin and Azithromycin.

C) Campylobacter G.E

- The infection is usually a self-limited but the illness is prolonged. The diarrhoea persists for more than a week in 1/3 of the children. Hydration with ORS is the only treatment needed in most cases.
- Anti diarrhoeal drugs may lead to prolongation of infection or perforation of the intestine and should not be used.
- Serve infections many require the use of antibiotics. Erythromycin and Azithromycin are the drugs of choice in children, both given orally. For systemic infection Amino glycosides can be given I.V.

D) **E.coli G.E**

- E.coli G.E is a self-limiting disease which usually settles in 1-3 days. If it is endemic, no treatment is required except hydration with ORS for the child who can take oral fluids and I.V. fluids otherwise.
- Traveler's diarrhoea may require antibiotic treatment. The most suitable antibiotics are: Trimethoprim/ sulfamethoxazole, Ciprofloxacin, Cephalosporin, Nitrrofurantoin and Amoxicillin.

E) **Yesrina G-E**

- Un complicated case of Yesrina G-E does not benefit from antibiotic therapy, but children with septicaemia or infection in sites other than the gastro intestinal tract should be treated with antibiotics.
- Patients with Yersina infection can be treated as outpatients but those who are dehydrated or have severe abdominal pain suggesting appendicitis and those with underlying disease like thalassemia should be hospitalized.
- Antibiotics used in Yersiniosis include: Gentamycin, Chloramphenicol, Cefotaxime, Ceftriaxone and Trimethoprim/ Sulfamethoxazole.

(3) Parasitic gastro enteritis

A) **Giardiasis**

- Giardiasis is a worldwide infection caused by Giardia lamblia. It is one of the most common water borne disease found both in drinking water and recreational water. Once a person or an animal is infected, the parasite lives in the small intestine blocking nutrients absorption and is detected in the stool.
- The infection is transmitted by faecal-oral route. Patient become infected when drinking contaminated water, eating contaminated uncooked food or accidently swallow Giardia picked up from surfaces contaminated with faces from infected person or animal.

- Those who are at risk of developing the infection are children in day care centres, travelers, children of infected parents and swimmers who swallow water of swimming Poole.
- Clinical presentation: Most people are asymptomatic and only 1/3 show symptoms. Symptoms could be acute or chromic.
    - Acute symptoms develop 1-2 weeks after ingestion of the cysts of Giardia. These include watery diarrhoea, flatulence, belching, abdominal cramps and pains, fever, nausea and occasionally vomiting. The illness is usually self limited, lasting for 2-6 weeks but may recur or become chromic
    - Chromic symptoms include loss of appetite, weight loss, lethargy, growth retardation, and enteropathy. The chromic disease is usually seen in those with immune deficiency syndromes.
- Diagnosis is by stool microscopy for the presence of giardia lamblia trophozoites and cysts. At least 3 stools should be collected on different days. The diagnosis can be made readily by examining the upper small intestine directly either by duodenal biopsy or through aspiration of jejunal contents or the string test (Entro –Test).
- An ELISA test (Enzyme- Linked Immunosorbent Assay) and counterimmuno electrophoresis of either stool or serum is available and has a deduction rate of 90%.
- Treatment of giardia infection: Metronidazole and Nitazoxanide are the drugs of choice.
  Metroniazole dose is 5mg/kg (up to 250mg) t.d.s. for 5 days; it has 80-90% efficacy.

  Nitazoxanide dose is 100mg (5ml) b.d. for 3 days for children aged 1-4 years, and 200mg (10ml) for children aged 4-11 years. Furazolidone has also been used.

- Prevention: avoid drinking unfiltered and untreated water and avoid eating uncooked foods that might have been washed with contaminated water. Drinking water should be boiled for at least 10 minutes if it has a risk of contamination.

B) Entamoeba Histolytica

- Amebiasis is world wide in distribution affecting 10% of the world's population mainly in the tropical areas and underdeveloped countries. It is the third commonest cause of death from parasitic infection after malaria and schistomiasis. Humans are the only reservoir for E.histolytica.
- Transmission is usually faecal- oral. Food and water become contaminated with cysts of E. histolytica. The cysts enter the small intestine and release the trophozoites which invade the large intestine epithelial cells causing flaks-shaped ulcers. The infection can spread from the intestine to the liver, lungs, brain, spleen etc via the venous blood.
- clinical manifestations of amoebiasis:
    - 90% of E.histolytic infections are asymptomatic. These are the carriers that pass cysts in their stools. The remaining 10% produce the disease which could be:
    - Acute amebic colitis which start with 1-2 weeks history of lower abdominal pain, watery diarrhoea containing blood and mucous, flatulence and tensmus. On abdominal examination, there will be tenderness on lower abdomen with palpably thickened large bowel. There may be low grade fever and dehydration.
    - Chromic amebic colitis: these present with recurrent episodes of bloody diarrhoea that wax and wane with alternating periods of constipation. The condition continues for months or even years.
    - Fulminant Colitis: this is an unusual presentation of amebiasis that is associated with 50% mortality rate. The child who is usually younger than 2 years or malnourished present with high fever, severe abdominal pain and profuse bloody diarrhoea. Dehydration and electrolyte abnormalities occur.
    - Amoeboma: Rarely there may be a localized amebic infection presenting as a tender abdominal mass in the Rt I iliac fossa

- Complications of amoebiasis: There could be intestinal or extra intestinal

  a) Intestinal complications:
  - Intestinal perforation and peritonitis are the most common.
  - Appendicitis.
  - Perianal ulcers: these are painful ulcers that usually respond to treatment.
  - Colonic strictures may develop after, colitis.

  b) Extra intestinal complications of amoebiasis
  - Amoebic liver abscess is the commonest extraintestinal form of amoebiasis, occurring in 1% of infected persons. It characteristically presents with:
    * Fever, right upper quadrant abdominal pain and tenderness. The pain may radiate to the right shoulder and laterally to the chest. Respiratory distress may develop. Patients usually give no history of significant gastro interstitial symptoms.
    * Examination may show hepatomegaly in 50% of the patients but jaundice is a rare finding. The patient may be anaemic and had lost Wt. Chest examination may reveal rales, decreased breath sounds and a friction rub.
    * The liver abscess may rupture into the pleural cavity causing pleuro- pulmonary amoebiasis or into the peritoneal cavity causing peritonitis or rarely into the pericardium causing pericarditis.
  - Lung abscesses may occur from haematongenous spread.
  - Cerebral amoebiasis may infrequently develop (haematogenous spread)
  - Genito urinary amoebiasis is a rare complication resulting from ruptured liver abscess, haematogenous spread or lymphatic spread.
- Diagnosis of amoebiasis
  - Stool examination for trophozoites is the diagnostic test for E.histolytica. 3 fresh specimens of stools (examined less than 20 minutes of collection) will give positive results in 90% of cases.

- ELISA assay for antigen detection and the indirect haemagglutination test for antibody detection are 95%positive for amoebic liver abscess and invasive amoebic colitis. These tests do not distinguish between acute and post infections.
- Barium study is contra indicated because of the risk of perforation.
- Ultrasound, CT and MRI scans of the abdomen are useful in diagnosing liver abscess. They can guide needle aspiration of the abscess for drainage and to obtain specimen for diagnosis
- Treatment: All symptomatic and asymptomatic patients who have E.histolytica trophozoites or cysts should be treated.
  - Asymptomatic patients are treated with Diloxanide furoate (20mg/kg/day)in 3 divided doses for 10 days or with Paromomycin (25-35mg/kg/day in 3 divided doses for 7 days)
  - Symptomatic patients with intestinal disease and hepatic abscess are best treated with Metronidazole in a daily dose of 50 mg/kg for 10 days in 3 divided doses, or Tinidazole in a daily dose of 50mg/k/day for 3 days Erythromycin is effective against intestinal amoebiasis but not hepatic abscess. Chloroquine is effective against hepatic amoebic abscess not intestinal amoebiasis

(4) Antibiotic-associated colitis

- Children who take antibiotics often develop diarrhoea (up to 60%). This is due to eradication of normal gut flora and overgrowth of other organisms.
- In most cases the condition is mild. Children present with watery diarrhoea but no other associated systemic symptoms. The diarrhoea decreases when the antibiotic therapy is stopped.
- A small group of patient, about 0.2-10% has pseudo membranous colitis, caused by toxins produced by clostridium difficile. This is usually seen after cephalosporin, amoxicillin and clindamycin. The diarrhoea may begin after several days of antibiotics exposure.

- Patients with pseudo membranous colitis present with abdominal pain, fever, diarrhoea and tensmus. The stool contains leukocytes and sometimes frank blood. WBC is often greater than 15,000. C. difficile toxin can be identified in the stool
- If C. difficile colitis goes unrecognized or untreated, complications may develop including toxic megacolon, perforation and peritonitis. Treatment is with oral Metronidazole (30 mg/kg/day) or oral Vancomycin (30-50 mg/kg/day) for 7 days. Relapse after treatment may occur and will require re-treatment with the same drug.

(5) Food Poisoning

Food poisoning is best defined as a gastrointestinal upset resulting in nausea, vomiting and diarrhea, with or without fever and appearing within 72 hours of ingestion of food contaminated by microorganisms or toxins. Usually other members of the family are affected. The likely offending agent varies according to the nature and time of onset of symptoms after the ingestion.

- Nausea and vomiting followed by diarrhoea. Onset within 1-6 hrs.
    1. Staphylococcus aureus toxins (food source: poultry, salads, milk)
    2. Bacillus cereus (Food source: fried and boiled rice, corn flour)
- Abdominal cramps and diarrhea. Onset within 8-16 hrs.
    1. Clostridium perfringens (source: red meat and poultry)
    2. Bacillus cereus (source as above)
- Fever, abdominal cramps, diarrhea within 16-48hrs
    1. Salmonella (source: eggs, poultry, beef, milk, salads)
    2. Shigella (source, salads and food contaminated by handlers)
    3. Vibrio parahaemolyticus (contaminated water and food)
    4. Invasive E. coli
    5. Campylobacter jejuni (poultry, milk)
- Abdominal cramps, watery diarrhea within 16-72hrs
    1. Enterotoxigenic E.coli
    2. Vibrio parahaemolyticus

3. Vibrio cholerae, Non 01
   4. Vibrio cholerae 01 (endemic area)
- Fever, abdominal cramps within 16-48hrs
   1. Yesrina enterocolitis
- Nausea, vomiting, paralysis within. 8-36hrs
   1. Clostridium botulinum
- Food poisoning occurs by two mechanisms:
   1. First, contamination of foodstuff by toxins or bacteria is the most common cause of poisoning. Foods in this case may either intrinsically contain toxins that manifest themselves under certain conditions (e.g. fish poisoning) or foods may become contaminated by bacterial or chemical toxins.
   2. Second, ingestion of intrinsically poisonous food stuffs may occur (mushroom poisoning is the example)

A) Salmonella food poisoning

- This is the commonest cause of food poisoning in the developing world. The highest attack rate occurs in young children with a peak between 6 months and 2 years.
- High protein foods such as poultry, meat, eggs and milk are most commonly associated with salmonella food poisoning. Some outbreaks were caused by contaminated chocolate bars and cold roast beef.
- The bacteria are easily killed by normal cooking temperature. Also if salmonella is present on raw or cooked food its growth can be controlled by refrigeration in below 40 F.
- The incubation period is 16-48 hrs. Diarrhoea is the commonest presenting symptom and it is usually severe and is often bloody. Headache, fever and chills may occur. Vomiting and abdominal pain are less prominent features. The illness last for 3-5 days. In neonates and immuno compromised patients the infection is complicated by bacteremia and meningitis.
- Treatment is by adequate hydration (ORS or I.V. fluids) as salmonella infection is a self limiting illness. Antibiotics are not needed for gastrointestinal symptoms because they prolong the carrier state and may cause replace in children. In neonates

and patients with bacteraemia or meningitis, Chloramphenicol, Cefotaxime or Ceftriaxone should be given.

B) Staphylococcal food poisoning

- Staphylococcus aureas from the respiratory tract, skin or superficial wounds may contaminate food (uncooked and poorly refrigerated) and produce toxins which will cause staph food poisoning if swallowed. Although cooking destroys the bacteria, the toxin produced is heat stable.
- Milk and milk products are the most common source of staph. food poisoning. Other common causes include salads containing egg and potatoes, sandwich spread, meat and poultry.
- Outbreaks occurred mainly due to food that has been cooked but left in room temperature for more than 4 hours or attributed to staph. carrier's food handlers. Cream-filled baked food account for 50% of the outbreaks.
- The incubation period is 1-6 hours. The diseases usually start with nausea abdominal pain and vomiting. The diarrhoea develops afterwards. The illness is self-limiting, recovering in 48hours. Death is very rare in this illness.
- Treatment is supportive with adequate hydration. Parenteral rehydration may be required in severe cases or for small infants with marked dehydration.

C) Bacillus cereus food poisoning

- Bacillus cereus is found in dust, soil and spices. It is an unusual cause of food poisoning. It may exist in spores whish are heat resistant.
- The source of the infection is usually starchy foods as rice, macaroni and potatoes. Outbreaks have resulted from the ingestion of contaminated Chinese food, lamb and vegetables.
- The illness results either from the ingestion of preformed toxins or from colonization of the gastro intestinal by the organism which produce toxins that activate intestinal adenyl cyclase causing secretary diarrhoea.
- Treatment is not required as symptoms are mild and self-limiting.

D) Clostridium Outline food poisoning

- Clostridium botulinum is an unusual cause of food poisoning but it is important because it causes death in up to 30% of cases and it occurs in home canned food or in infant's honey.
- The organism produces an extremely potent neurotoxin. These could be preformed toxins or result from ingestion and gastro intestinal colonization with toxin producing strains as the cases in infants. The toxin blocks the presynaptic release of acetylcholine.
- The canned food may show signs of spoilage such as bulging can and off odour. Boiling of food for 10 minutes or heating at 80C for 30 minutes before eating will destroy the toxin.
- In infants younger than 6 month, the initial symptoms are severe hypotonia and constipation. The infant will have week cry and poor sucking, pooled oral secretions, cranial nerves palsy and generalized weakness.
- The incubation period is 8-36 hours in older children. Symptoms start with nausea, vomiting, lethargy and headache. The patient will then have the classical tried of a) No fever, b) Symmetrical flaccid descending paralysis with bulbar palsies (dysphagia, dysphonia, dysarthria and diplopia). C) Clear sensation. Death results from respiratory failure.
- Diagnosis is made by finding C. botulinum toxin in stool, serum or vomitus of the patient. The EMG will show the characteristic pattern of BSAP (brief, small, abundant motor-unit action potentials)
- Treatment is with antitoxin or passive human botulism immune globulin which should be given as soon as the clinical diagnosis is made.

E) Clostridium perfringes food poisoning

- This is a rather common cause of food poisoning (3d commonest in UK and USA) Meat and gravy are the typical sources of the infection. Following the ingestion of contaminated foods, the organism multiply in the small intestine and produce toxins which cause the symptoms.

- The incubation period is 8-16 hours. The illness present with abdominal cramps and diarrhoea. Vomiting and fever are unusual. The illness is self-limited resolving within 24 hours. Most of the infection is a subclinical and patient forms antibody against the toxin.

F) **Vibrio parahaemolyticus**

- This is an unusual cause of food poisoning resulting from ingestion of raw or undercooked seafood. The infection can also be transmitted by faecal-oral route.
  The organism invades the intestinal mucosa as well as producing a haemolysin which causes the clinical disease.
- The incubation period is 16-72 hours. The illness presents as explosive watery diarrhoea, nausea, vomiting, abdominal cramps and sometimes fever. It is self-limited resolving in 1-3 days.
- Treatment is not required expect in severe cases when fluid and electrolyte replacement is indicated.

(6) Non-gastrointestinal (Parenteral)

- Upper respiration tract infection may present with diarrhoea, e.g.tonsilitis
- Systemic infections may cause diarrhoea e.g. UTI, pneumonia, Otitis media
- The symptoms of the localized infection will be more evident than diarrhoea.

(7) Surgical Conditions

- Intussusception may present with diarrhoea (5% of cases) but the spasms of screaming with colic, drawing up of legs and pallor predominate. The infants appear comfortable between the attacks. They pass current jelly stools mixed with blood and mucous.
- Acute appendicitis can present as acute diarrhoea. Fever, vomiting and acute abdominal pain are prominent symptoms. Abdominal

tenderness with a positive rebound tenderness point to the diagnosis of acute appendicitis.
- Necrotizing Entrocolitis may present with bloody diarrhoea in the early stages of the disease together with vomiting and abdominal distention. It occurs in preterm babies, usually in the second week after birth. It is the commonest neonatal surgical emergency.

(8) Congenital Chloride diarrhoea

- This is a genetic disorder due to autosomal recessive mutation on chromosome7
  It causes persistent secretary diarrhoea which starts during foetal life leading to polyhydramnios and premature delivery.
- The watery diarrhoea continues after birth leading to dehydration, abdominal distension with visible peristalsis and failure to thrive. There will be hypoelectrolytaemia and hyperbilirubinaemia. The stool chloride is >90mmol/l
- Treatment is by early correction of dehydration and replacement of NaCl and KCl. This will result in normal growth and development.

[II] CHRONIC DIARRHOEA

(1) Chronic Gastroenteritis

- Chronic Giardiasis can cause chronic diarrhoea. Symptoms include loss of appetite, weight loss, lethargy, growth retardation, and enteropathy. The chronic disease is usually seen in those with immune deficiency syndromes.
- Amoebiasis may present as chromic amebic colitis with recurrent episodes of bloody diarrhoea that wax and wane with alternating periods of constipation. The condition continues for months or even years.
- HIV infection and other immunodeficiency disorders can present with chronic diarrhoea.

(2) Post Gastroenteritis diarrhoea

- Sometimes a return of watery diarrhoea occurs with the introduction of normal diet after successfully treating gastroenteritis. This is usually due to temporary lactose intolerance.
- This can be confirmed by a positive clinitest of the stools due to the presence of sugars. Treatment is by return to ORS for a day or two before trying normal diet again. If no improvement a lactose free diet should be given for 1-2 weeks.
- Occasionally multiple dietary intolerance may result. This is treated by a food free of cow's milk, disaccharidases and gluten for two weeks before the reintroduction of normal diet.

(3) Toddler's Diarrhoea

- This is chronic non specific diarrhoea which is usually seen in children 1-4 years of age as watery stools, increased flatus and abdominal distension without other symptoms. These children usually drink too much juice but they have normal appetite and they grow and develop normally.
- The condition usually settles after reducing the fluid intake and increases the amount of fibre and fat in the diet.

(4) Cow's milk and soya protein intolerance

- Cow's milk protein may cause an immune-mediated inflammatory reaction in the small intestinal mucosa leading to the development of villous atrophy. This is seen in about 7% of all infants, with preterms at an increased risk.
- These infants present with diarrhoea which may show blood and mucous, baby colic, vomiting and anaemia. The diagnosis is suspected when symptoms develop after introduction of cow's milk.
- The skin prick allergy test and RAST test may be helpful in making the diagnosis. Small intestinal biopsy will help in making the diagnosis. Confirmation of the diagnosis is when the symptoms disappear on removal of cow's milk and recur when it is reintroduced.

- About 30% of children with cow's milk intolerance are also sensitive to soya protein. These children develop similar symptoms that are seen with cow's milk allergy. Treatment for these children is by giving goat's milk (Golden Goat) or camel's milk to older infant.

(5) Malabsorption Syndromes

- There are many causes of malabsorption during childhood. The common causes include: cystic fibrosis, coeliac disease, mono and disaccharidases deficiency, inflammatory bowel disease, lymphangiectasis, Abeta- lipoproteinaemia, pancreatic insufficiency and bile salts deficiency.
- Early manifestations of malabsorption syndromes include frequent bulky foul smelling stools. There is an associated failure to gain weight in spite of the initially good appetite. Abdominal distention follows.
- Quantitative assessment of fat absorption is done by measurement of fat excreted in stools in 3 days as proportion of fat intake(infants should not excrete > 15% and children only 5% of their total fat intake), stool pH and reducing substances will test carbohydrate malabsorption.
- Special tests for specific malabsorption include: sweat chloride test for cystic fibrosis, intestinal mucosal biopsy for coeliac disease, Giardiasis, inflammatory bowel disease, lymphangiectasis and a betalipoproteinaemia. Barium study can be helpful in inflammatory bowel disease.
- Blood tests for serum iron, ferritin, LFTs, Ca, phosphates, serum folic acid, B12, and immunoglobulins will help in assessing specific malabsorption.

(6) Lactose & Fructose intolerance, Sucrase-isomaltase deficiency

- Deficiency of the enzyme lactase leads to lactase intolerance with development of diarrhoea, abdominal pain, bloating and weight loss after taking milk and other dairy products. It is common

among Asians and Africans. Lactase enzyme supplements reduce the symptoms.
- Fructose is the sugar found in many fruits. Many children develop diarrhoea after taking fructose. Treatment is by avoiding fructose rich foods.
- Sucrase and isomaltase deficiency is the commonest form of disaccharidase deficiency occurring in infancy. It is inherited as autosomal recessive. The diarrhoea begins with the introduction of sucrose containing food.

(7) Inflammatory bowel disease

- This includes Crohn's disease and Ulcerative colitis. Diarrhoea is most common presentation, usually containing blood and mucous. There will be weight loss due to malabsorption, lethargy, fever and anaemia.
- The abdomen is distended and tender. There may be perianal abscesses, skin tags, fissures or fistulae. Skin rashes (erythema nodosum and pyoderma gangrenosum) and arthritis may be present
- WBC, ESR, CRP are raised. Albumen, iron, folic acid and vit B12 are reduced. Barium enema can be helpful in the diagnosis. Colonoscopy and biopsy will confirm the diagnosis and determine the extent of the disease.

(8) Irritable bowel syndrome

- It is usually seen in older children with a prolonged history of intermittent diarrhoea alternating with constipation and normal bowel motions. These patients have cramps aching abdominal pain which is localized in the lower abdomen over the sigmoid colon and is eased by passing stool or flatus.
- The diagnosis is one of exclusion.

(9) Vitamin B3 (Niacin) deficiency

- Deficiency is rare but causes Pellagra which presents with: high sensitivity to sunlight, poor appetite and weight loss, ataxia,

weakness, aggression and the 5d's of dermatitis, diarrhoea, depression, dementia and death if not treated within 5 years.
- Also folate deficiency may present with diarrhoea. There will be megaloblastic anaemia.

(10) Tumours (gastroenteropancreatic neuroendocrine tumours)

- These are carcinogenic tumours between the endocrine system and nervous system. The majority of these are carcinoids and pancreatic endocrine tumours.
- Diarrhoea or increased number of bowel movements is one of the presenting symptoms, usually due to increased hormonal secretion.

(11) Chemotherapy and Radiation therapy diarrhoea

- Most chemotherapy may kill some intestinal cells or cause injury leading to the development of temporary diarrhoea which disappears when the drug is stopped.
- Radiation therapy may cause diarrhoea within one week if the intestine is in the treatment field. The radiation causes injury to the intestinal mucosa affecting the absorption.

(12) Endocrine causes

- Addison's disease commonly present with fatigue, muscle pains & weakness, diarrhoea, vomiting sweating, fever and hyperpigmentation. BP, blood sugars and serum Na are low while serum K is high. Metabolic acidosis develops.
- Hyperthyroidism may also present with diarrhoea. Signs of the disease will be noted.

(13) Acrodermatitis Entropathica

- This is a rare disorder inherited as autosomal recessive. The basic defect is impaired intestinal absorption of zinc leading to severe systemic deficiency.
- The average age of onset of symptoms is 9 month after weaning of breastfeeding. The earliest sign is usually fissures at the angle of the month and the perioral rash which then spread to the face and behind the ears. The rash also appears in the distal extremities, knees and trunk as vesiculobullous lesions
- Diarrhoea and steatorrhea then develop, with or without vomiting. Irritability is seen in infants and emotional disturbances in older children including depression, apathy and paranoia. Alopecia develops preceded by the hair being sparse, brittle and reddish in colour. Treatment is with Zinc sulphate.

(14) A beta Lipoproteinaemia

- This is an inborn error of lipoprotein metabolism, which is inherited as autosomal recessive. Symptoms and signs appear in the first few months of life as diarrhoea with fatty, pale, frothy stools. There is failure to thrive due to malabsorption, primary degeneration of the retina, muscle weakness, ataxic neuropathy, scoliosis and mental retardation.
- The RBC show abnormal shapes (Acanthocytosis), The total cholesterol is below 70 mg/dl, the triglycerides and low-density lipoproteins are undetectable.
  There is deficiency of Vit A, Vit D, Vit E and VitK.
- Treatment is with large amounts of Vit E and dietary restriction of triglycerides.

(15) Intestinal lymphangiectasis

- Lymphangeciasis is the abnormal dilatation of the lymphatic vessels. Congenital malformation of the lymphatics is the commonest cause of it.

- Chronic diarrhoea is always the presenting feature. There is also vomiting and loss of weight. The blood shows low lymphocyte count, reduced serum proteins, low calcium level and low cholesterol.

(16) Laxative abuse

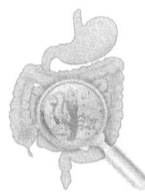

MALABSORPTION SYNDROME

- These are disorders affecting the digestion and absorption of nutrients.
- Early manifestations of malabsorption are:
    - Abnormal stools which are frequent, bulky, foul-smelling and are difficult to flush down the toilet.
    - Failure to gain weight
    - Good appetite initially
- Late manifestations are
    - Wight loss
    - Muscle wasting especially buttocks
    - Distended abdomen
    - Specific nutrient deficiencies, either singly or in combination
    - Reduced immunity secondary to certain nutrient deficiency

Causes of Malabsorption syndrome are numerous. They include:

1- Abnormal structure of the gastro intestinal tract (reduced digestion/absorption)

  a/ Gastric resection with or without dumping syndrome
  b/ Malrotation
  c/ Stenosis of jejunum or ileum
  d/ Small bowel resection / short bowel syndrome
  e/ Multiple polyposis interfering with absorption

2-Pancreatic insufficiency (causing reduced digestion)

    a / Cystic fibrosis
    b /Shwachman syndrome
    c/ Chronic pancreatitis
    d/ Pancreatic pseudo cysts
    e/ Enterokinase, lipase and co lipase deficiency
    f/ Pearson syndrome
    g/ Malnutrition

3-Bile salts deficiency (causing reduced digestion)

    a/ Neonatal hepatitis
    b/ Biliary atresia
    c/ Acute and chronic active hepatitis
    d/ Cirrhosis of the liver

4-Intestinal abnormalities (causing reduced absorption)

    a/ Mucosal disease
        -Infection: Viral and bacterial
        -Infestation: Giardiasis, Hookworm, Tapeworm
        -Malnutrition
    b/ Cow's milk and soy protein intolerance
    c/ Coeliac disease
    d/ Secondary Mono and Disaccharidase intolerance
    e/ Dermatitis Herpetiformis
    f/ Tropical sprue
    g/ Crohn's disease
    h/ Familial villous atrophy
    I / Aids

5-Selective inborn absorptive defects

    a/ Glucose-galactose malabsorption
    b/ Primary disaccharidase deficiency
    c/ Hereditary fructose intolerance
    d/ Cystinuria, Methionine malabsorption

e/ Hartnup disease
f/ Congenital malabsorption of folic acid
g/ Selective malabsorption of vit B12
h/ Zinc malabsorption in Acrodermatitis enteropathica
i/ Congenital chloridorrhoea
k/ Abetalipoproteinaemia
l/ Primary hypomagnesemia
m/ Familial hypophosphataemic rickets

6) Vascular and lymphatic disease

a/ Intestinal lymphangiectasis
b/ Lymphoma
c/ Whipple disease
d/ Congestive heart disease
e/ Scleroderma

7) Other Causes

a/ Radiation enteritis
b/ HistocytosisX
c/ Renal failure
d/ Immune deficiency disorders
e/ Drugs e.g. antibiotics, Neomycin, Methotrexate
f/ Wolman disease

- Diagnosis depends on the history of disease with time of onset of symptoms, detailed dietary history, family history and associated symptoms. Careful examination looking for general signs of malabsorption and specific signs for special causes might give a clue to the diagnosis.
- Investigation will include:
    • Stool examination for blood, WBC, fat contents, pH and reducing substances. Stools are also tested for parasites.
    • Quantitative assessment of fat absorption is by measurement of fat excreted in stools as a proportion of fat intake after collection of stool for 3 days. Infants should not excrete

more than 15% of their fat intake while older children will excrete only 5% of their total fat intake.
- Fat malabsorption may show decreased levels of Vit A, Vit E, 25 hydroxy cholicalciferol (Vit D) and prothrombin time.
- D-Xylose test will give an assessment to the carbohydrate absorption by intestinal mucosa.
- Lactose and sucrose malabsoption can be measured by the breath hydrogen technique. There will be increased breath hydrogen after ingestion of carbohydrate
- Accurate assessment of protein absorption is difficult. It requires isotopic labeling of amino acids. But, protein loosing enteropathy can be estimated by measurement of fecal α-1-antitrypsin.
- Blood tests including liver function tests, serum iron and ferritin, Ca, Phosphates, alkaline phosphates, serum folic acid, serum B12, renal function and immunoglobulins will be of help in assessing specific causes of malabsorption
- Special tests for specific causes of malabsorption include: Sweat chloride test for cystic fibrosis, intestinal mucosal biopsy for coeliac disease, giardiasis, inflammatory bowel disease, lymphangiectasia and abetalipo- protinemia.
- Barium study can be helpful only in inflammatory bowel disease and may show a non specific small intestinal malabsorption pattern.

Disorder of disaccharide absorption

- Disaccharidase enzymes are present at high level in the jejunum and in the proximal ileum. They act on the dietary disaccharides and the oligosaccharide products of pancreatic amylase action on starch before significant absorption can take place.
- Deficiency of disaccharidase can be primary (congenital) or secondary (acquired)

- Primary congenital disaccharidase deficiency is rare. These include:

Congenital lactose deficiency which is a rare condition leading to:
- Diarrhoea after lactose is ingested and stools are frothy and acid
- Vomiting is common
- Malnutrition may occur
- Stools are positive for reducing substances and have low pH.
- There is a rise in breath hydrogen after oral administration of lactose.
- Lactose tolerance test can be done in which the blood glucose fails to rise more than 10mg/dl after ingestion of 1g of lactose
- Dietary starch and sucrose tolerance is normal
- Patient with lactase deficiency respond to reduction of dietary lactose. For older children lactase- containing tablets can be ingested to reduce symptoms when taking lactose containing diets.
- Genetically determined lactose deficiency may develop after age 3-5 years in same racial groups.
- Congenital Sucrase and isomaltase deficiency is the most common form of disaccharides deficiency occurring in infancy
    - ❖ It is inherited as an autosomal recessive
    - ❖ It present as diarrhoea that begins with the introduction of sucrose-containing foods or drinks.
    - ❖ Vomiting may occur
    - ❖ Abdominal distention and bloating is common
    - ❖ Failure to thrive may develop
    - ❖ Children develop reluctance to take food containing sucrose.
    - ❖ Reducing substance in stools may be negative because sucrose is not reducing sugar.
    - ❖ Diagnosis may be confirmed by elevated breath hydrogen after ingestion of sucrose.
    - ❖ A sucrose tolerance test may be abnormal
    - ❖ Stool chromatography may be diagnostic.

- Jejunal mucosal biopsy will show deficiency of the enzyme
- Treatment is by elimination of foods that contain more than 2% of sucrose.

-Secondary (Acquired) Lactase deficiency

- This often occurs as a result of damage to the small intestinal mucosa following severe viral gastro enteritis.
- The condition is transient and is usually self limited lasting for days or at most weeks after the gastro enteritis settles.
- Mucosal recovery occurs fully in about 4 weeks.
- Other causes of secondary lactose deficiency include all condition that lead to intestinal mucosal injury e.g. coeliac disease, giardiasis, malnutrition, abeta- lipoproteinaemia etc.
- Patients present with the characteristic loose explosive stool
- Reducing substances in the stools are positive
- Stools chromatography may be diagnostic
- Breath hydrogen is elevated after done looking after ingestion of lactose
- Small intestinal biopsy done looking for the underlying cause will show reduced activity of lactase.

-Secondary sucrase deficiency

- It is caused by all conditions that lead to intestinal mucosal damage.
- Signs of sucrase deficiency are usually masked by the more striking symptoms of lactase deficiency which is seen in the intestinal mucosal injury

Monosaccharides malabsorption (Glucose-Galactose malabsorpion)

- Primary glucose – galactose malabsorption is a rare autosomal recessively inherited condition. The Na-glucose transport protein is defective.

- The abnormal gene is localized to the long arm of chrmosme22.
- There will be severe impairment of the transport of glucose in the intestinal epithelium and renal tubular epithelium.
- Rapid onset of watery diarrhoea is noticed from birth. This responds to withholding glucose& galactose and relapses on reintroduction
- Reducing substances in stools are positive and the pH is acidic.

Glycosuria may be present

- Small bowel biopsy and disaccharidase estimation are normal
- The glucose tolerance test is flat
- Treatment is by giving fructose as the main carbohydrate source
- The acquired (secondary) glucose-galactose malabsorption is seen in infants with gastro-enteritis. Here both the disaccharides and monosaccharides are malabsorped

  The disaccharides and monosaccharides are malabsorped temporary. The condition is self limited.
- The prognosis for glucose – galactose malabsorption is good because tolerance improves with age.

Cow's milk protein intolerance

- The cow's milk protein may cause an immune- mediated inflammatory reaction in the small intestinal mucosa with the development of villous atrophy. The exact immune mechanisms are undetermined but the clinical spectrum of the intolerance includes:
  - Acute type 1-mediated hypersensitivity
  - Delayed onset hypersensitivity
  - Cow's milk sensitive enteropathy
  - Cow's milk allergic colitis
  - Other non specific symptoms that might be attributed to cow's milk
- Milk protein intolerance is more common in males than females
- There is usually a family history of atopy.

- About 7% of all infants are intolerant to cow's milk. Premature infants are at an increased risk.
- The major symptoms are due to enterocolitis features leading to:
    - Baby colic
    - Vomiting
    - Diarrhoea
    - Blood and mucous in stools
    - Anaemia
    - Sigmoidoscopic examination and rectal biopsy reveal superficial colitis with eosinophilic infiltration and lymphonucliar hyperplasia.
- Less commonly, protein loosing enteropathy may develop due to eosinophilic gastro enteritis. The clinical features include:
    - Prolonged diarrhoea that begins by 2-3 month of age
    - Hypoalbuminaemia with development of oedema.
    - Hypogammaglobulinaemia\
    - Weight loss
- Small intestinal villous atrophy manifestations may develop causing
    - Malabsorption syndrome
    - Hypoalbuminaemia
    - Passing blood in stools
    - Anaemia later in childhood
- Rarely anaphylactic shock may be a manifestation of cow's milk allergy. This is a life threatening condition which should be assessed under supervision by experienced clinicians.
- Sometimes breast fed infants may develop similar symptoms to cow's milk allergy and the elimination of whole cow milk from the mother's diet may cause disappearance of those symptoms.
- For diagnosis of cows milk allergy, the skin-prick allergy testing and RAST test may be useful.
- Confirmation of the diagnosis is when the attributable symptoms disappear on removal of cow's milk protein and recur when it is reintroduced.
- Small intestinal biopsy will help in confirming the diagnosis.
- About 30% of children with cow milk intolerance are also sensitive to soy protein. These patients develop similar symptoms that are seen with cow's milk protein intolerance.

- Treatment of patients with cow's milk protein is by total elimination of cow's milk from their diet. These infants are fed with hydrolysed protein formula, like Nutramigen, Pregestimil, and Prejomin. These protein are broken down into oligopeptides and peptides.
- Most patients with Cow's milk protein allergy will eventually tolerate normal diet by 2-3 year of age.

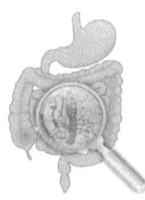

COELIAC DISEASE

- Coeliac disease is an entropathy resulting from intestinal sensitivity to the gliadine fraction of gluten in wheat, rye, barley & oats.
- It is thought to be a cell- mediated immune reaction to gliadine which leads to the intestinal damage and villous atrophy.
- The incidence of coeliac disease varies, in different parts of the world, between 1 in 250 and 1 in 3000. The use of serological screening tests has shown a higher incidence of asymptomatic cases.
- There is an increased incidence of the disease in children with diabetes, Down syndrome, 1gA deficiency, thyroiditis and individuals with HLA-DR3 and –DR4
- Early presentations of coeliac disease are:
    - Diarrhoea or abnormal stools which start after the introduction of gluten in the diet, usually between 6-18 month of age. The stools with time become bulky and foul smelling
    - Irritability and a miserable looking infant
    - Anorexia associated with failure to gain weight.
    - Abdominal distension and buttock wasting
- Late presentation of coeliac disease (seen in older children)
    - Iron deficiency anaemia
    - Rickets and osteomalacia
    - Short stature and delayed puberty
- Unusual presentation include
    - Peripheral oedema
    - Finger clubbing

- A triad of Constipation, Vomiting and Abdominal pain
- Folate deficiency
- Asymptomatic coeliac disease has been detected on screening programs using serologic assays.
- Diagnosis of coeliac disease will start by general investigations to show the malabsorption features. These include:
    - D-xylose test will show impaired absorption of the D-xylose with blood levels less than 20 mg/dl, one hour after ingestion.
    - Fat contacts of the stools after 3 days collection will show increased fecal fat. Values more than 15% of the daily fat intake are suggestive.
    - Serum Iron will show low levels in older children.
    - Serum protein will show hypoalbuminaemia in some cases.
    - The whole blood foliate level is usually low.
    - Elevated serum level of antigliadine, antireticulum and Endomysial antibodies.
    - X-rays of the bones of hand and forearm or legs may show evidence of rickets in an old child or osteoporosis.
    - Brain study will show a malabsopative pattern.
- Confirmatory test of coeliac disease is small intestinal biopsies. An initial jejunal biopsy will show villous atrophy, partial or total followed by a second biopsy, taken after administration of a gluten-free diet, showing impairment. Rarely a third biopsy showing reappearance of the disease after gluten challenge may be needed.
- Screening tests for coeliac disease is done by antihuman transglutaminase antibody assay, or Endomysial antibody test. These are the most sensitive and specific screening tests. Both are of the 1g A class, so patients who are 1g A deficient may give false negative results. The anti- endomysial antibody will turn –ve in a child with coeliac disease on gluten free diet.
- Treatment consists of elimination of dietary gluten for life. Improvement is expected within a week. The patient should be given a well balanced diet supplemented with vitamins and minerals. The small intestinal mucosa will show recovery within 3-12 month.
- Coeliac crises can be seen in very ill patients as follows:
    - Severe diarrhoea

- Profound malnutrition
- Abdominal distension
- Peripheral oedema
- Acidosis
- Dehydration
- shock
- Steroids are given to patients in coeliac crises as well as correction the dehydration and the electrolyte in balance.
- Malignant lymphoma of the small bowel and other gastro intestinal malignancies may occur in long standing cases of coeliac cases if the diet is not adhered to.

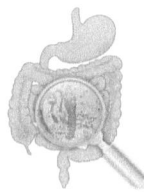

CYSTIC FIBROSIS

- This is the most common genetic disorder of the white population
- It is a multisystem disorder with a wide spectrum of clinical manifestations including gastrointestinal.
- The most common and serious manifestations of CF are the respiratory ones which are:
    - Persistent cough which is usually the first symptom.
    - Recurrent chest infection.
    - Recurrent wheezing suggestive of asthma
    - Purulent sputum with or without haemptysis in old children.
    - Nasal polyps and chronic sinusitis
    - Allergic Bronchopulmonary Aspergillosis (ABPA) i.e. allergy to Aspergillus fumigatus.
    - Clinical signs may show Harrison sulci, barrel shaped chest, downward displacement of the liver and finger clubbing.
- The gastrointestinal manifestation of C.F. includes:
    - Meconium ileus causing intestinal obstruction in up to 15% of neonates with C.F.
    - Distal intestinal obstruction syndrome (DIOS) or meconium ileus equivalent occurring in older children.
    - Malabsoption syndrome with bulky offensive stools in about 90% of pts.
    - Recurrent rectal prolapse in 10% of patients
    - Failure to thrive in spite of the very good appetite
    - Atresia of the bowel occurs with increased frequency in patient with C.F.
    - Pancreatic insufficiency in most patients

- Exocrine pancreatic insufficiency with abnormal glucose tolerance in 10% of patients.
- Diabetes mellitus occurs with increasing frequency after the age of 10 years
- Inadequate absorption of fat soluble vitamins may lead to:
  ❖ Bleeding disorders due to Vit. K deficiency
  ❖ Benign intracranial pressure caused by Vit A deficiency
  ❖ Haemolytic anemia and neurological symptoms due to Vit E deficiency
- Serve hypochloraemic metabolic alkalosis caused by salt deficiency
- Hepatic abnormalities of C.F include:
  ❖ Prolonged neonatal jaundice
  ❖ Hepatomegaly due to fatty liver
  ❖ Focal biliary fibrosis
  ❖ Liver cirrhosis and portal hypertension in some adolescents.
  ❖ Variceal haemorrhage with haematemesis.
  ❖ Cholelithiasis and obstruction to bile duct
- There is an increased incidence of gastrointestinal malignancies among cystic fibrosis patients.

− Other presentations include: short stature, male infertility, head exhaustion and Pseudo-Barter's syndrome
− The diagnosis of C.F. can be confirmed by sweat test and or genetic testing.
  - Sweat chloride test >60 m mol/l is considered diagnostic of C.F
  - Sweat chloride of 40-60 m ml/l is considered highly suggestive of C.F. In such situation the sweat test should be repeated or genetic testing should be done.
  - Genetic DNA testing for C.F. Tran membrane regulator (CFTR) is used as a diagnostic test.
  - Neonatal screening using radioimmunology assay for immunoreactive trypsin has been used in newborns. The immunoreactive trypsin (IRT) is raised in the first few weeks of life in babies with C.F. Confirmation with DNA analysis should be done for raised IRT.

Acrodermatitis Enteropathica

- This is a rare disorder inherited as autosomal recessive.
- The basic defect is impaired intestinal absorption of zinc leading to severe systemic deficiency. The clinical features are:
- The average age of onset is 9 month. Children who are breast-fed are detected later, after weaning, as breast milk has more bioavailable zinc.
- The earliest sign is usually fissures at the angle of the month and the perioral rash which then spread to the face and behind the ears.
- Perianal rash develops, initially erythematous rash then become psoriatic-like plaques.
- Rash also appears in the distal extremities, knees and trunk as vesiculobullous lesions
- Diarrhoea and steatorrhea with or without vomiting
- Irritability in infants and emotional disturbances in older children including depression, apathy and paranoia.
- Alopecia preceded by the hair being sparse, brittle and reddish in colour.
- Repeated bacterial infection and monilia infection.
- Ocular manifestations including photophobia, conjunctivitis and corneal dystrophy.
- Paronychia and nail dystrophy are also seen in some patients.
- Neurological features like tremor, ataxia may be seen.
- Poor wound healing may be noticed.
- Serum zinc and alkaline phosphate are low in the blood. Hypolipoproteinaemia may be detected. Blood ammonia is elevated.
- Dramatic improvement to zinc therapy proves the diagnosis.

Familial chloride Diarrhoea

- This condition is inherited as autosomal recessive.
- There is profuse watery diarrhoea that may begin in utero.
- There is often a history of polyhydramnios.
- The diarrhoea begins at birth and the stools resemble urine.

- There is usually abdominal distension. Ileus may develop due to hypokalameia.
- Characteristically the serum sodium and chloride are low.
- The stool Chloride is high as well as the stool PH.
- There is hypochloraemic, hypokalaemic metabolic alkalosis
- Infants are anorexic and lethargic.
- Failure to thrive develops in the early days of life.
- Treatment is by giving sodium and potassium chloride supplements.
- Early diagnosis and early treatment make the prognosis good.

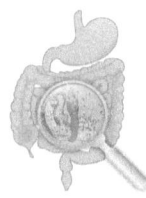

DEHYDRATION

- Morbidity and mortality in gastro enteritis are caused primarily by water and electrolyte losses. Therefore the key to the management is the prevention of dehydration and promotion of rehydration in those already dehydrated
- Infants are at particular risk of dehydration because:
    - Their greater surface to weight ratio leading to greater insensible water losses (about 15-17 ml/kg/day)
    - Their basal fluid requirement is high (100-120ml/kg/day) which is10-12% of their body weight.
    - Their renal tubular reabsorption process is immature and cannot compensate for the losses.
    - They cannot reach for fluids when they are thirsty.
- Types of dehydration
    1- Isotonic dehydration when sodium and water lost are in proportion to each other. Serum Na is 130-150 mmol/L.
    2- Hyponatraemic dehydration when proportionately more sodium is lost than water. Serum Na is <130mmol/L.
    3- Hypernatraemic dehydration when proportionately more water is lost than sodium. Serum Na is >150mmol/L. Clinical signs of dehydration here are less prominent. The features of dehydration are mainly doughy feel to the skin with or without irritability and fever. Weight change remains the most reliable indicator of dehydration degree. Seizure occurs in severe cases.
- In all three types there is usually a total body deficit of salt and water.

- If the illness is acute i.e. illness less than 3 days, 80% of fluid loss is from the extracellular fluid (ECF) and 20% from the intracellular fluid (ICF). ECF contain mainly Na at 140 mmol /L and ICF contains K at 150 mmol/L.
- Management of dehydration depends on the accurate estimate of the level of dehydration and the type of dehydration. Hypoglycaemia may complicate dehydration.
- Estimation of severity of dehydration depends on the accurate estimate of the level of dehydration and the type of dehydration.
- Estimation of severity of dehydration is done by:
    1-Weight loss as a percentage of total body weight prior to the dehydration episode. But accurate weight immediately pre-illness is rarely available in clinical situation.
    2-Clinical signs of dehydration:
- This is widely to asses the degree of dehydration. Dry oral mucosa, decreased skin turgor, sunken eyes and altered neurological status are probably the best clinical signs correlating with dehydration.
- Also decreased peripheral perfusion (capillary refill time) and deep acidotic breathing are good clinical signs. A high blood urea and low blood pH are positive tests associated with dehydration.
- The presence of 2 or more of: capillary refill time >2 seconds, absence of tears, dry mucous membranes and ill appearance suggest dehydration of at least 5%.
- The following table could be used:

Sign/symptom	Mild <5%	Moderate	Severe	Notes
-Wt loss	<5%	5-10%	>10%	<ul><li>Watery diarrhoea may make nappies appear wet.</li></ul>
-Dry month and mucous membranes	+/-	+	++	<ul><li>Mouth breathers are always dry.</li><li>Malnourished and marasmic children will have decreased skin turgor.</li></ul>
	-	+/-	+	

Sign	No dehydration	Some dehydration	Severe dehydration	Notes
-decreased skin turgor		+/-		
-Neurological status	Normal	Restless or lethargic	Drowsy	
-Tears	Reduced	Absent	Absent	
-Eyes	Normal/slight sunken	Sunken	Very sunken	
-Anterior fontanelle	Flat	Sunken	Very sunken	• Anterior fontanelle will be closed by 18 month of age
-Urine output	Decreased	Reduced	Marked oliguria	
-Tachycardia	-	-/+	+	
-Tachyponea	-	+-/+	+	• Hypovolaemia, fever and irritability cause tachycardia
-Capillary refill time	Normal	Prolonged	>2seconds	• Metabolic acidosis and pyrexia make tachypnoea worse
-BP	Normal	Normal	v. low or un-recordable	

- The following factors in history of a child presenting with diarrhoea should alert the clinician to a high risk of significant dehydration:
- Infants less than 6months of the age for the reasons mentioned earlier.
- More than 8 significant diarrhoeal stools in the last 24 hours
- More than 8 significant vomits associated with the diarrrhoea in the last 24 hrs. (A significant vomit is anything more than effortless small volume regurgitation)
- General recommendations for children presenting with acute gastroenteritis:
    - Children who are severely dehydrated should be admitted to hospital.
    - Children with moderate dehydration should be observed in the paediatric facility of the hospital for at least 6 hours to ensure successful rehydration (3-4 hours) and maintenance of hydration (2-3hours).

- Children at high risk, mentioned earlier, should be in a hospital paediatric facility for at least 4-6 hours to ensure adequate maintenance of hydration.
- Children whose parents are thought to be unable to manage the child's condition at home successfully should be admitted to hospital.

— Management of mild dehydration:-
- Should be managed by short term substitution of maintenance fluid, a suitable glucose-electrolyte solution (ORS). This may be rice-based. Small amounts are given more frequently.
- The solution is given until vomiting and profuse diarrhoea subsides, usually lasting less than 24 hours.
- Normal diet can then be introduced immediately.

— Management of moderate dehydration:
- The estimated deficit of 6-10% should be replaced with ORS (60-100mls/kg) over a period of 3-4 hours. Small amounts are given more frequently. It is recommended to be given as 5 ml measures every 1-2 minutes. If this is well tolerated with no vomiting the amount can be increased with decreasing the frequency. Over night rehydrate by continuous naso-gastric tube infusion.
- Regularly assess success of rehydration every two hours. If no improvement in clinical signs of dehydration or worsening signs, consider naso-gastric tube infusion or intravenous infusion.
- After replacement of deficit, the child should be offered his normal maintenance. This is calculated as follows:

Body weight	Fluid requirement per day	Fluid requirement per hour
First 10kg.	100 ml/kg	4ml/kg
Second 10kg.	50 ml/kg	2ml/kg
Subsequent kg (Remaining kg of body weight).	20ml/kg	1ml/kg

- The ongoing losses should be replaced with 10ml/kg of ORS for each loose stool and substantial vomit.
- To prevent recurrence of dehydration after full hydration, the child should be allowed unrestricted fluids either milk or water.
- Rapid introduction of feeding following rehydration reduces the duration of illness and the number of loose stools as well as improving nutrition.
- Breast feeding children should continue to breast feed through the rehydration and maintenance phases of their acute illness.
- If the dehydrated child with gastro-enteritis is normally formula fed, feeds should stop during rehydration and restart as soon as the child is rehydrated (4hours).

- Type of ORS used should be suitable with the type of dehydration.
  - The WHO ORS which contains 90 mmol/L of sodium is suitable in developing countries where rapid loses of sodium and potassium are documented (hyponatraemic cholera like diarrhoea) The osmolarity of WHO ORS is 311 mmol/L.
  - In developed countries, diarrhoea tends to be isotonic so replacement of large amounts of sodium is not suitable and may be harmful. In such cases ORS with 60 mmol/L sodium and osmolarity of 224 mmol/L is suitable.
  - ORS is contraindicated in altered mental status with risk of aspiration, abdominal ileus and underlying intestinal malabsorption.
  - To reduce the incidence and frequency of vomiting an antemetic like Ondansetron (Serotonin Receptor Antagonist, 5-HT3)may be given to improve the success of oral hydration and help avoid IV fluid therapy.

- Management of severe dehydration is by I.V. fluids as follows:
  - Blood should be taken for electrolytes and bicarbonate as well as urea, creatinine and haematocrit with WBC.
  - If the child is shocked, he will need rapid IV infusion to restore circulation and renal perfusion. 20 ms/kg of normal saline or ringer lactate given over 15 minutes. In severe dehydration a second bolus of 20ml/kg should be given., up to 60ml/kg may be needed within 1 hour.

- The child will then need fluids for replacement of fluid deficit + maintenance.
    ❖ Fluid deficit may be calculated as follows:
    Percentage of dehydration X Weight in kg X 10 = fluids in mls.
    ❖ Maintenance fluid is calculated as 100 mls/kg for first 10 kg, 50 mls/kg for the second 10 kg and 20mls/kg for subsequent kg.
- The I.V fluid used is 0.45% saline in 2.5-4% dextrose
- The plasma sodium result should decide the rate of infusion:
- In patients with low or normal sodium, lost fluid can be replaced over 24hrs. 1/2deficit + 1/3 of maintenance in the first-8hs. The rest are given in the remaining 16hrs.
- In hypernatraemic patients (Na>150mmr/l) fluid must be replaced over at least 48 hours and sometimes longer depending on the severity, the higher the sodium the slower the rehydration must be. Too rapid reduction in plasma sodium will lead to a shift of water into cerebral cells resulting in cerebral oedema and possible convulsions and death.
Aim to bring down the serum Na in hypernatraemic patients by 5 mmol per day. ORS, if possible, is quicker in the correction of dehydration and acidosis and is safer than I.V. therapy.
- Potassium deficit is corrected, after urine has passed, in 48 hours. 1/2 k deficit is corrected in each day of the first 2 days not exceeding 40mmol/L.
- Patients with disturbed electrolytes should have their plasma electrolytes checked 4 hourly.
- Children with fever may require extra 1 ml/kg per degree centigrade every hour in addition to maintenance therapy.
- After restoration of circulating fluid volume, further rehydration can be done orally with ORS given small amounts more frequently, if the patient is stable and the mental state allows.
- Following rehydration, there should be rapid introduction of feeding. This will reduce the duration of illness and the number of loose stools. Breast fed infants should continue

to breast feed through the rehydration and maintenance phases while formula fed infants should stop feeds during rehydration and restart as soon as the infant is rehydrated.
- Infants and children with acute gastro-enteritis should not be treated with anti-diarrhoeal agents. They are ineffective, may prolong the excretion of bacteria in stools and are associated with side-effects. They might also focus the attention away from oral rehydration.
- Children with gastro-enteritis are recommended to have stool culture in the following conditions:
    o A history of blood with or without mucous in stool.
    o When the child is systemically unwell, have severe or prolonged diarrhoea.
    o A history suggestive of food poisoning.
    o When there is abrupt onset of diarrhoea with more than 4 stools per day and no vomiting pre-diarrhoea.
    o When the patient is admitted to hospital.

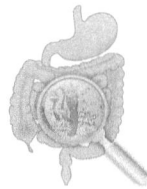

DEFECATION DISORDERS

Constipation

- Breast-fed infants commonly pass 4-5 stools a day but some breast-fed infants may not pass stools for several days. This is all normal.
- Normal infants often strain while passing normal stools up to the age 3 months. This may wrongly be considered as constipation.
- Constipation is passing hard or bulky dry stools infrequently.
- In children, constipation often follows on acute fibrile illness, dietary changes, a superficial anal fissure, a psychological family stress or the used of disliked WBC at school or on holiday. In such cases constipation is only temporary and is resolved with appropriate diet.
- A detailed hostory about stool consistency, frequently of defecation duration of constipation, dietary habits, family history as well as careful abdominical and rectal examinations is essential to reach an accurate diagnosis.
- The causes of constipation includes:
    1. Normal Variation
        - Breast-fed infants
        - Normal habit
    2. Functional
        - Forceful toilet training
        - Psychological stress
        - Dislike for school bathrooms or on holiday
        - Anorexia Nervosa
        - Hot weather/ insufficient fluid intake.

3. Dietary causes
    - Dehydration
    - Malnutrition
    - Excessive milk intake
    - Lack of bulk
4. Painful defecation
    - Anal Fissure
    - Proctitis
    - Perianal Abscess
    - Rectal prolapse
    - Rectal polyps/ Haemorrhoids
    - Sexual Abuse
    - Foreign body
5. Drugs
    - Lead
    - Narcotics
    - Anti-depressants
    - Viricristine
    - Excess use or overdose of laxatives, (causing pain)
    - Antihistamines
6. Mechanical Obstruction
    - Hirschsprung disease
    - Waardenburg Syndrome
    - Rectal Stenosis
    - Anal Stenosis
    - Anterior Ectopic Anus
    - Meconium ileus equivalent
    - Pelvic masses / small bowel masses
    - Chronic volvulus/ intussusception
7. Hypo and hyperganglionosis
    - Von Recklinghausen Disease
    - Multiple endocrine neoplasia
    - Intestinal neural dysplasia
8. Endocrine causes/ Metabolic causes
    - Hypothyroidism
    - Hyperparathyroidism
    - Hypercalcaemia
    - Hypermagnesaemia

- Hypokalaemia
- Diabetis Insipidus
- Renal tubular acidosis
9. Neuromuscular disease/ Smooth Muscle disease
    - Hypotonia/ Down Syndrome
    - Werdnig-Hofman Disease
    - Cerebral Palsy
    - Myotonia/ Muscular dystrophy
    - Infantile Botulism
    - Abscent Abdominal Muscles (Prune Belly's Syndrome)
    - Chagas disease
    - Spinal Cord disease
    - Scleroderma/ dermatomyositis
    - SLE
    - Complications of Constipation include:
        o Distention of the rectum with decrease of rectal sensation for urge of defecation.
        o Abdominal pain due to impacted faeces.
        o Overflow diarrhea due to leakage around the faecal mass.
        o Rectal bleeding
        o Anal Fissure caused by the passage of hard bulky stools.
        o Urinary Track Infection due to pressure on the urethra.
        o Encopresis
- Treatment of constipation will involved the following steps:
    o Dietary modification by:
        ▪ Increase fluid intake i.e. water, juices
        ▪ Add fruits and vegetables to diet
        ▪ Add fiber food like Bran, whole wheat
        ▪ Use of Barley malt extract as Maltsupex 5 mls t.d.s added to feed.
    o Stools softener such as dioctyl, naturacil, hydrocil, lactulose
    o Stimulant laxatives like Senekot maybe needed.
    o Lubricants such as castor oil, mineral oil twice/ day.

- o Impacted rectum should be cleared of impacted stool by use of enema like fleet enema 1oz/10kg. Glycerine suppository may be of help.
- o Anal fissures and absces should be dealt with appropriately. Vaseline ointment or vasogen help small fissures.
- o Toilet training like sitting in a time for bathroom in the morning after a drink and also after meals. Education for patients and parents is important.
- o Specific underlying aetiology should be treated appropriatelty.
- o Encouragement by family and health prifessionals is essential as well as using a reward system to prevent relapse.

Encopresis

- This is soiling by formed stools beyond the age of expected toilet training at 4-5 years. This is more common in boys than girls.
- Encopresis frequently cause emotional, social and family problems.
- It could either be involuntary overflow soiling or voluntary non-overflow incontinence.
- The involuntary overflows soiling form the majority of the cases. The hard massive retained faeces breakdown allowing the uncontrolled passage of foul smelling liquid stools from the rectum.
- The voluntary soiling often indicates the presence of significal psychological problem in the child or family. There is usual and associated problems of enuresis.
- As encopresis is a complication of constipation, the underlying aetiology is the same. The earlier in life the problem of defecation occurs the more likely an organic pathology is the underlying causes.
- Detailed histoty with stress on the method of toilet training, social history, diet and presence of painful defecation together with careful abdominal examination feeling for palpable faecal matter and rectal examination confirming the presence of hard stool in the rectum. In Hirschsprung disease the ompula may be empty.
- For most children where underlying pathology is not suspected. No investigation is required. If Hirschsprung disease is suspected or

there is voluntary soiling or failed medical treatment the following investigation maybe done:
- o Baruim enema. It shows distended rectum infunctional constipation but a narrow distal segment with proximal megacolon in Hirschsprung disease.
- o Rectal manometry. It will show normal relaxation of the internal sphincter with normal recto anal reflex in functional constipation. In hirschsprung disease there will be no sphincter relaxation.
- o Rectal biopsy will show normal ganglion cells present in functional constipation but abscent ganglion cell in Hirschsprung disease.

– Treatment of encopresis should start with emptying the rectum of any retained faeces to allow normal tone to return to the distended rectum. Repeated rectal washout may be needed. Other treatments used for constipation will also be applicable to encopresis with stress on the training programme.

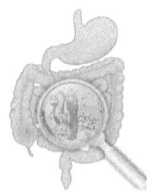

ACUTE ABDOMINAL PAIN

- Acute Gastroenteritis
- Urinary Tract Infection
- Appendicitis
- Mesenteric adenitis
- Pneumonia
- Constipation
- Sickling corses
- Trauma to the abdomen
- Intussuseption
- Intestinal obstruction
- Milk intolerance
- Neprotic Syndrome
- Peritonitis
- Meckel's Diverticulitus
- Volvulus Malrotation
- Parazitic infection
- Pelvic infection
- Crohn's Disease
- Ulcerative Colitis
- Henoch- Schonlein Purpura
- Hepatitis
- Pancreatitis
- Cholecysititis
- Gall Bladder stone
- Tortion of testis
- Epididymitis
- Tortion of ovarian pedicle

- Obstructive hernia
- Diabetic ketoacidosis
- Addisonian crises
- Battered baby syndrome
- Lead poisoning
- Familial Mediterranian fever
- Porphyria
- Rheumatic fever/ Mycocarditis/ Pericarditis
- Renal Calculi
- Tumors

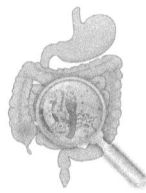

ACUTE HEPATITIS

- Acute viral hepatitis can be caused by the hepatitis viruses A, B, C, D, E.
- Most of the infectious with hepatitis viruses are asymptomatic.
- Indeveloping countries, most children are exposed to HAV by age 10 years but onlu 20% are exposed by age 10 years in developed countries.

Hepatitis A

- It is RNA viruses transmitted by faecal-oral route either by contact with affected patients or as an epidemic from contaminated food or water. Rarely it is transmitted through blood to a neonate.
- The incubation period is 15-40 days
- Hepatitis AV typically causes minor illness in children with more than 80% of cases being asymptomatic.
- The initial symptoms are non-specific including fever, anorexia, abdominal pain, headache and vomiting followed by dark yellow urine. 5-10 days later, the jaundice develops. The jaundice lasts 1 to 4 weeks usually.
- Blood shows raised conjugated and unconjugated serum bilirubin, high ESR or normal WBC. The liver enzymes transanemiasis are raised. The alkaline phosphatase is also raised.
- A positive IgM antibody indicates an acute illness which IgG anti HAV persists after recovery. Lifelong immunity to HAV develops.
- 99% of children recover completely. Rarely fulminating hepatitis may develop in 0.1% of the cases. This is due to massive hepatic

necrosis. The jaundice deepens, encephalopathy develops and coma may occur. The transaminasis fall which the prothrombin time becomes marked by prolong. Other serious prognostic marker are hypoalbuminemia, hypoglycaemia, and an elavated gammaglobulin praction > 2.5 g/dl.
- Few patients with HAV develop prolonged cholestatic hepatitis with jaundice remaining for few months, but it is self limiting.
- A benign relapse of symptoms may occur in some patients after 6-10 weeks of appearant resolution.
- Rare cases of aplastic anemia following HAV have been reported.
- Treatment: There is no specific treatment and no evidence that bed rest or change of diet is effective.
- Prevention is by passibe and active immunization.
    o Passive immunization is with immune globulin 0.02-0.04ml/kg I.M. for exposed subject within 1-2 weeks of exposure. It gives up to 90% prevention, but last for 3-6 months.
    o Active immunization is with HAV vaccine.

Hepatitis B Virus

- HBV is transmitted by vertical transmission to infants from their mothers who are carriers. The discase is also caused later in life from blood products, needles prick, skin tattoos, renal dialysis or through sexual transmission. Breast milk and saliva are shown to contain viral antigen, explaining the high incidences.
- The incubation period is 21-135 days of infection in family contacts.
- HBV is a DNA virus compost of core antigen called HbcAg, which is found in the nucleus of infected liver cells, and a double outer shell surface antigen called HbsAg. There is an envelop (e) antigen system that appears in the serum of infected patients early and correlates with active virus replication. It is called HbeAg. Its presence is a marker of infectivity. Antibodies to all the 3 antigens will be produced by the human body in response to these antigens.
- Children with HBV are usually asymptromatic but some have classical features of acute hepatitis. Visible jaundice is the main sign followed by dark coloured urine. Hepatomegaly may be

- present and to less degree spleanomegaly and lymphadenopathy may be present too.
- An illness resembling serum sickness occurs before the appearance of jaundice in about 10% of the patients. This presents with maculopopular rash, urticaria and arthritis affecting knees, elbows, wrists and ankles.
- The majority of patients will resolve spontaneously, but 1-2% develop fulminant hepatic failure while 5-10% become chronic carriers.
- Rarely, patients with acute HB infection present with acute pancreatitis.
- The LFTs and haematology findings are similar to HAV.
- As diagnostic test for HBV, most centers use HbsAg (HB surface antigen and the antibosy against HbcIgm (IgM anticore). Persistence of HbsAg will indicate chronic infection.
- Infants infected from their mothers ususally become asymptomatic carriers. Approximately 30-50% of this will develop HBV liver disease which may progress to cirrhosis in 10%. There is a long term risk of developing hepatocellular carcinoma.
- Treatment of chronic HBV is unsatisfactory. Interferon, 5-6 million units/m2 body surface area 3 times a week for 4-6 months inhibits viral replication in only 30-40% patients and leads to the appearance of anti HBC. Asymptomatic HbsAg carriers may not respond. The new drug Lamivudine maybe more effective. Liver transplant.
- Prevention is by mass population with HBV vaccine. These are 3 dozes, the first is given at birth followed by the second dose at 1-2 months of age and the third dose 5-6 month later. Unvaccinated contacts are given HB immunoglobulin (HBIG) I.M. in a dose of 0.06ml/kg as soon as possible after exposure, up to 7 days. This is followed by giving the vaccination. Individuals at risk of developing HBV should be immunized.

Hepatitis C

- HCV is a single- stranded DNA virus which has atleast 7 genotypes.

- In children it is transmitted by unscreened blood or blood products especially patients with haemophilia and haemoglobinopathies. Vertical transmission from infected mothers occurs especially if mothers are HIV positive. Transmission of the virus from the breast milk is rare.
- The incubation period is 1- 5 month.
- Infection with HCV is usually asymptomatic but acute hepatitis can occur. At least 70 % develop chronic liver disease. Cirrhosis and hepatocellular carcinoma may occur after a number of years.
- Infected infants have elavated liver enzymes but do not appear ill. Their long term outcome is not known.
- Antibodies to hepatitis C appear relatively late in the course of infection.
- Screening test for hepatitis C virus infection use second generation ELISA test with recombinant viral antigens on patients serum. Confirmation is done by the radioimmunoblot assay (RIBA) or HCV RNA by PCR.
- Treatment of HCV in the acute stage is supportive. The chronic infection is treated by a combination of interferon. And ribavirin. Relapses are common. Patients in liver failure are treated by liver transplantation with good outcome. Reinfection may occure. There are no vaccine as yet for HCV.

Hepatitis D

- it is RNA virus which requires a coat pf HBV to become infectious.
- The incubation period is the same as HBV. It occurs as a co-infection with hepatitis B or as a superinfection causing an acute exacerbation of chronic hepatiits B virus infection.
- The transmission is parenteral and by intimate contact. Vertical transmission is rare.
- The infection can be asymptomatic or as an acute hepatitis. Fulminant hepatic failure is rare. Cirrhosis develops in 50-70% of there chronic infecitons.
- Diagnosis is by detection of anti HDV 1gM. Also HbsAG is detected.
- Treatment is by high dose of interferm toeradicate HBV.

Hepatitis E

- it is an RNA virus which is resopnsible for epidemic non A, non B hepatitis
- it is transmitted by fecal-oral route. It is seen in the developing countries due to water-born epidemics.
- The clinical course of hepatitis is similar to hepatitis A but sympotomatic disease is rare in children. It occurs in adolescents and adults.
- If it affects a pregannt woman in the third trimester the mortality is as high as 20%
- Diagnosis is suspeted when aetiology of viral hepatitis is not identified. Confirmation of diagonsis is established by detecting auto HEV.
- Complete recovery from acute infection of HEV occurs and chronic infection has not been described.
- There is no specific treatment for HEV
- There is no vaccine or proplylaxis treatment available.

Fulminant hepatic failure

- fulminant hepatic failure is uncommon in children but has high mortality (80%)
- it is defined as acute liver dysfunction resulting in hepatic coma and congulation defect within 6 weeks after the onset of the illness.
- It may occur in patients who have no pre existing pathology of the liver
- The causes of acute liver failure in children include:
    - In neonates the following may cause acute liver failure
        - Viral infections, namely herpes siplex, adenovirus and enteroviruses
        - Galactosemia
        - Fructose intolerance
        - Iyrosinaemia
        - Neonatal iron storage disease
        - Fatty acid oxidation defect
        - Familial histrocytosis

- Bile acid synthesis defects
  - in children the causes are
    - viral hepatitis: B, C non A-C, E and rarely A
    - poisons/ drugs: paracetamol, INAH, Halothane, poisonous mushroom
    - metabolic: Wilsoon's Disease, acute fatty liver
    - autoimmune hepatitis
    - HIV infection
    - Reye's Syndrome
- Clinical presentation is with increasing jaundice, hypoglycemia, electrolyte disturbances, irritablity, aggression, confusion and drowsiness, ascites and rapidly shrinking liver. Coma occurs hyperflexia and a positive extension plantar response may be seen. Fetor hepaticus breath odor will be noticed.
- Complication include: haemorrhage from gastritis due to coagulopathy, sepsis, pacreatitis, impaired renal fuunction and cerebral oedema.
- Diagnosis: there is high serum bilirubin, liver enzymes initially high but may decrease in the terminal stages, hypammonemia, hyploglycemia, low serum albumin, increased alkaline phosphatase, prolonged prothrombin time, blood urea is low. EEG will show acute hepatic encephalopathy and a CT scan may show cerebral oedema.
- Treatment is directed towards:
  - Maintaining normal blood sugar by IV dextrose
  - Preventing haemorrage with IV vitamin K, fresh frozen plasma even exchange transfusion which will also correct biochemisty temporary
  - Preventing sepsis with broad spectrum antibiotics
  - Sterlization of the gut by adding metronidazole or lactuloze to the antibiotics
  - Treating cerebral oedema by fluid restriction and mannitol diuretico
- Toxins should be removed if they are the causative organism. Plasmaphoresis and charcoal/ hemoperfusion maybe required N-acetylcysteine is the treatment for paracetamol poisoning.
- Lover transplant in patients with poor prognosis could be the only hope. It is successful in 60-85% of cases.

- Poor prognosis is associated with the following situation:
- Shrinking liver
- A rising biliruben > 20mg/dl following transminasis
- Prothrombin over 30 seconds and factor V levels <20%
- Progressing coma

Reye's Syndrome

- this is an acute non-inflammatory encephalopathy with microvescular fatty infiltration of the liver
- most case occur between 4 and 12 years of age with a peak at 6 years.
- There was a close associaion with aspriin therapy in epidemics of influenza A or B virus and varicella infections. The incidence of Reye's syndrome has dropped dramtically since stopping giving aspirin to chidlren with viral infections.
- The clinical manifestations are as follows:
    o Continuous vomiting during or immediately URTI. H/O aspirin therapy
    o Altered level of consiousness as confusion, aggittation then coma
    o No fever and no jaundice but liver may be palpable
    o The pupil are dilated, reflexes are exaggerated and acidotic breathing
    o CSF examination shows normal result.
- blood test shows: hypoglycemia, hyperammonemmia, acidosis, elevated transaminase and prolonged prothrombin time.
- Diagnosis is made on a liver biopsy which shows microvascular fatty infilteration without necrosis or inflammation
- Treatment is the sae as in fulminent liver failure.

Wilson Disease (Hepatolenticular Degeneration)

- this is an autosomal recesive inheritance. It is caused by a mutation in the gene on chromosme 13. It results in impared bile excretion

of copper and decrease in the plasma protein which tranports copper (caeruloplasma) (caeruloplasmin)
- ther will be accumulation of copper in the liver, eyes, brain, kideneys and bones. This will lead to the following clinical manifestation, usually after the age of 5 years old.
    o Liver: chronic active hepatitis with jaundice and hepatosplenomegaly, fulminant hepatits may occur. Portal hypetension and cirrhosis.
    o Eyes: Kayser-Fleischer rings and sunflowe cataract
    o Brain: deteriation of school performance, tremor, dysarthria personality and pyschiatric disorders.
    o Kidney: renal tubular acidosis and vitamin D resistant rickets
    o Blood: Haemolytoc anameia
- the diagnosis is suggested by low serum caeruloplasmin and copper. Normal serrum copper may be formed early in the disease but there will be high urinary copper excretion. Also glycosuria nad aminoaciduria may be detected.
- The blood test also show high serum bilirubin, haemolytic anaemia, decrease serum uric acid and low alkaline phosphatase in acute Wilson disease.
- Liver biopsy will show increase copper depositio. Mallory bodies can be seen.
- Treatment. To give D-penicillamine as a coper chelating agent, for life. Vitamin B6 supplements should be given to prevent optic neuritis. Food high in copper like chocolate, nuts and dried fruits should be avoided. Oral zinc interferes with copper absorption from the gut, so can be supplemened.
- The prognosis is good if treatment is started early otherweise the disease can be fatal.

Cirrhosis of the liver

- This is the end stage of many forms of liver disease, characterized histologically by:
    o diffuse hepatocyte injury
    o increase in connective tissue leading to irrevsible fibrosis

- o disorganization of the lobular and vasulcar architecture leading to portal hypertension
- o formation of regeneration nodles, which may be micronodular or macronodular
- The cause of cirrhosis are classified as:
    - o Biliary tract disorders
        - Bilairy artesia
        - Choledochal cyst
        - Common bile duct sterosis
        - Timors of the bile duct
        - Primary sclerosis cholengitis
        - Cyptic fibrosis
        - Caroli disease byler disease
    - o Infections
        - Viral hepatitis (B, C or Non A, B, C)
        - CMV
        - Neonatal giant cell hepatitis
    - o Autoimmune disease
    - o Drugs and toxins e, g cytotoxic drugs and alcohol
    - o Metabolic causes
        - Wilson disease
        - Alpha-I antitrypsin deficiency
        - Haemochromatosis
    - o Total Parenteral Nutrition TPN
    - o Inborn errors of metabolism:
        - o Galacto semia
        - o Fructose intoelrance
        - o Tyrosinaemia
        - o Glycogen storgae diseases
- Clinical manifestations of cirrhosis include:
    - o Palmar erythema
    - o Spider naevi
    - o Pruritus with cutaneous excoriation
    - o Failute to thrive
    - o Jaundice may be present
    - o Bruising easliy
    - o Anaemia
    - o Clubbing

- o Liver may be palpable depending on the udnerlying cause
- o Gastro intestinal hage
- o Ascites
- o Splenomegaly
- o Gynaecomastia in males
- o Peri orbital oedema
- o Encephalopathy
- Laboratory results depend on the uderlying cause but usually there is:
    - o Mild rise in liver enzymes
    - o Low serum albumen but raised gammaglobins
    - o Prolonged prothrombin time
    - o Haemolytoc anaemia with burr and target red cells
    - o Leuokopenia or thrombocytopenia
- liver ultrasound and CT scan may show the nodules and abnormal texture
- liver biopsy will show the regeneration nodules with surrounding fibrosis. Abnormalities of the biliary system will be noted:
    - o portal hypertension
    - o variceal bledding
    - o malnutrition
    - o increased susceptability to infections
    - o ascitis with or without peritonitis
    - o hepatocellular cercinoma
    - o hepatorenal sundrome (with renal failure)
    - o pulmonary hypertnesion
    - o hormonal disturbances
    - o impaired melatbolism of drugs and hormones
    - o encephalopathy
- treatment is towrds the underlying cause to stop progression of the disease. Transplantation of the liver may be the answer in some causes. A well balanced diet with adequate calorie intake and vitamins. Treat any complication.

Portal Hypertension

- It is defined as an increase in the portal venous pressure to more than 5mm Hg above the inferior vena caval pressure
- Causes of portal hypertension is classifies as follows
    1. Pre-hepatic causes due to (usually in infants who were previously healthy and with no liver disease
        a. Portal Vein thrombosis and splenic vein thrombosis caused by:
            - Neonatal omphalocitis
            - Umbilical vein catheterization
            - Dehydration
            - Sepsis / peritonitis / pancreatitis
        b. Portal Vein or splenic vessel malformations caused by
            - Atresia / stenosis x splenic artery aneurism
            - Valves
    2. Intrahepatic Causes
        a. Cirrhosis of the liver as a major cause of portal hypertension
        b. Veno-occlusive disease
            i. Complications of bone marrow transplant
            ii. Chemotherapy complications
            iii. Some herbal teas (bush tea) ingestion
            iv. Toxins in forms of food (India and Jamaica)
        c. Congenital Hepatic fibrosis (autosomal recessive inheritance)
        d. Schistosomiasis
        e. Hepatic Cyst
        f. Idiopathic portal hypertension (non-cirrhotic portal fibrosis
    3. Supra hepatic causes
        a. Budd-Chiari Syndrome
        b. Right ventricular failure
        c. Constrictive pericarditis
- Clinical findings of portal hypertension are as follows
    o Splenomegaly as the cardinal feature of portal hypertension
    o Ascites
    o Large tender liver in cases due to suprahepatic causes
    o Jaundice may be present depending on underlying cause

- - -
  - o Failure to thrive
  - o Increased incidence of infection / hypoalbuminaemia
  - o Distended superficial veins on the anterior abdominal wall and back
  - o Caput medusa with flow of blood from umbilicus and venous hum above the umbilicus
  - o Hemorrhoids
  - o Eosophageal varices causing haematemesis and melena
  - o Anaemia
  - o Hypersplenism causing thrombocytopenia and granulocytopenia
  - o Impaired coagulation
  - o Uncontrolled gastrointestinal haemorrhage exaggerated by thrombocytopenia and impaired coagulation
  - o Encephalopathy
- Special Investigations include:
  - o Upper endoscopy looking for eosophageal varices
  - o Liver biopsy
  - o Doppler ultrasound for liver, portal, splenic and hepatic veins as well as inferior vena cava
  - o Angiography will be diagnostic in non hepatic causes.
- Treatment is mainly towards management of the complication of portal hypertension namely:
  - o Blood transfusion to replace blood loss
  - o Vasopressin infusion on to reduce portal pressure and flow by constricting the splenic arterioles
  - o Endoscopic sclerotherapy for bleeding eosophageal varices
  - o Portosystemic shunt operations to decompress the portal system
- Liver Transplantation may be needed n certain cases

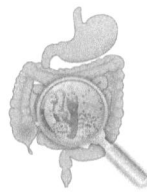

LIVER TRANSPLANTATION

- Liver Transplantation has revolutionized the prognosis for children with end-stage liver failure
- Indications for liver transplant include:
    o Chronic liver disease patients who have severe malnutrition, failed to thrive and develop in their milestones or with recurrent complications and poor quality of life
    o Extrahepatic biliary atresia is the most frequent indication
    o Metabolic disorder: Wilson disease, Alpha-1 anitrypsin deficiency, tyrosinaemia, galactosemia, Criggler-Wajjar Syndrome Type 1
    o Fulminant Hepatic Necrosis
    o Autoimmune chronic active hepatitis, hepatitis B & C
    o Liver malignancy (some)
- Contraindication to liver transplant include: Sepsis, untreatable cardio-pulmonary disease or cerebrovascular disease
- Up to 85% of children survived for at least 5 years so far.
- Most children receive part of an adult liver as it is difficult to obtain a small liver for the children
- Post transplant immunosuppression involves prednisone + cyclosporine or tacrolimus. Azathioprine is sometimes used.
- Complications post-transplantation include:
    o Primary graft failure (non-function of the liver)
    o Hepatic artery thrombosis
    o Infection. Septicaemia is the main cause of death
    o Biliary leaks and strictures
    o Graft rejection
    o Lymphoproliferative disease caused Epstein-Barr virus

Acute Pancreatitis

- Acute pancreatitis is caused in children due to:
    o Infection mainly viral including: EBV, mumps, Coxsackie virus, hepatitis A, B and HIV. Also bacterial like B-haemolytic streptococcus and salmonella
    o Trauma to the abdomen, usually blunt or penetrating including surgery
    o Obstruction to pancreatic flow from any cause like tumors, duplications, ascaris, congenital duodenal stenosis
    o Biliary tract disease as: cholelithiasis, choledochal cyst
    o Systemic diseases as: SLE, Cystic fibrosis, diabetes, Crohns disease, Henoch-Schonlein purpura, Kawasaki disease, chronic renal failure Type 1 and V
    o Genetic condition: Cystic fibrosis, Shawachman syndrome, Pearson syndrome
    o Metabolic diseases: Glycogen Storage disease, hyperlipidemia, Reye syndrome, Alpha-1 Antitrypsin deficiency, Hypercalcaemia, organic acidopathies or during rapid feeding in cases of malnutrition
    o Drugs: Sulfasalazine, Azathioprine, Thiazides, Valproic acid, Alcohol in teenagers and high dose corticosteroids
    o Idiopathic in 20% cases
- Clinical manifestations include:
    o Abdominal pain in the most consistent symptoms, usually upper or mid-abdominal. It may radiate to the back and is classically constant and knife-like.
    o Vomiting is a common symptom
    o The abdomen is tender but not rigid and bowel sounds are diminished
    o Ascites and left sided pleural effusion may be present
    o Other associated physical findings depend of the aetiology and the development of complications
    o Poor prognostic signs are periumbilical bruising (Cullen's sign) and bruising on the flanks (Grey Turner's sign) both indicating haemorhagic pancreatitis
- Blood tests show raised serum amylase and also serum lipase which persists longer than the amylase. There may be elevated

WBC, hyperglycemia with blood sugar usually 7200mg/ dc, rising urea and acidosis but low serum albumin, haematocrit and hypocalcaemia. Lactate dehydrogenase is elevated.
- Plain X-ray abdomen, abdominal ultrasound and CT scan may be needed to evaluate the extent of the disease. Endoscopic retrograde cholongiopancreatoduedenoscopy (ERCP) and MRCP may be requires in some cases.
- Complications of acute pancreatitis include:
    o Shock and electrolyte disturbances
    o Ileus with features of intestinal obstruction
    o Acute respiratory distress syndrome
    o Hypocalcaemic tetany
    o Gastrointestinal haemorrhage
    o Pancreatic pseudo cyst which usually resolves spontaneously but rarely may rupture or get infected.
    o Pancreatic abscess formation is a rare complication
    o Chronic pancreatitis
    o Malabsorption due to pancreatic insufficiency
    o Diabetes mellitus
- Treatment is mainly medical including fluid replacement, bowel rest, nasogastric decompression, analgesics like morphine, parenteral nutrition and broad spectrum antibiotic. Surgical treatment is reserved for cases caused by trauma.

Causes of Hepatomegaly

1) Infections

    a. Viral
        - Hepatitis A
        - Hepatitis B
        - EBV
        - Chronic Active Hepatitis
    b. Bacterial
        - Typhoid
        - Tuberculosis
        - Brucellosis

- Sepsis/Liver abscess
- Rocky mountain spotted fever

c. Parasitic
- Malaria
- Schistosomiasis
- Leishmaniasis
- Amoebiasis
- Hydatid disease
- Ascariasis
- Toxocariasis

d. Protazoal
- Babesiosis (in USA)
- Liver flukes
- Leptospirosis

e. Fungal
- Histoplasmosis

2) Blood Disease
- Haemolytic anaemias (sickle cell, Thalassemia, spherocytosis)
- Iron deficiency anaemia
- Leukemias and lymphoma
- Familial Erythrophagocytic lymphohistiocytosis

3) Storage / Metabolic Disorders
- Galactosemia
- Glycogen storage disease
- Alpha-1 antitrypsin deficiency
- Disorders of the Urea cycle
- Mucopolysaccharidosis
- Hereditary fructose intolerance
- Generalized Gangliosidosis (Type 1)
- Fucosidosis
- Lipidosis
- Homocystinuria
- Haemochromatosis
- Amyloidosis

- Hypervitaminosis
- Hyperlipoproteinemia

4) Drugs and Toxins
    - Acetaminophentoxicity
    - Phenobarbital
    - Sulfonamides
    - Tetracycline
    - Corticosteroids

5) Tumours / Malignancy
    - Hepatoblastoma
    - Wilms Tumour
    - Hepatocarcinoma
    - Neuroblastoma
    - Haemangioma of liver
    - Histiocytosis X (Letterer-Siwe Diseases
    - Metastatic Tumours
    - Hamartomas

6) Vascular
    - Budd-chiari Syndrome
    - Congestive Heart Failure
    - Constrictive pericarditis
    - Rendu-Osler-Weber Syndrome (hereditary Hemorrhagic Telangiectasia)

7) Congenital
    - Congenital Hepatic Fibrosis
    - Familial Intrahepatic cholestasis
    - Zellweger Syndrome
    - Wolman Disease
    - Farber disease
    - Multiple Sulfatase deficiency
    - Moore-Federman Syndrome
    - Hand-Schuller-Christian disease
    - Chediak-Higashi Syndrome
    - Beckwith-Wiederman Syndrome

8) Miscellaneous
   - Cystic Fibrosis
   - Obesity
   - Starvation
   - Veno-occlusive disease
   - Reye's Syndrome
   - Pseudohepatomegaly (liver displaced down)
   - Acquired Immune deficiency syndrome
   - Juvenile Rheumatoid arthritis

Causes of Splenomegaly

1) Infections

   a. Viral Infections
      - EBV
      - CMV
      - Rubella
      - Herpes Simplex
   b. Bacterial
      - Severe Pneumonia (usually stephylococeal)
      - Septiceamia
      - Bacterial endocarditis
      - Typhoid
      - Brucellosis
      - TB
      - Tularemia
      - Plague
      - Splenic abscess
   c. Parasitic
      - Malaria
      - Schistosomiasis
      - Leishmeniasis
      - Toxocariasis
   d. Protazoal
      - Trypanosomiasis

- Babesiosis
- Toxoplasmosis
    e. Spirochaetal
        - Leptospirosis
    f. Fungal
        - Histoplasmosis
        - Coccidiodomycosis

2) Blood Diseases
    a. Congenital haemolytic aneamia (Thalassaemia, Sickle cell anaemia, H6C Spherocytosis, Ellyptocytosis, Stomatocystosis, Pyruvate Kinase Disease, G-6-P-D deficiency
    b. Isoimmunization due to blood group incompatibility
    c. Autoimmune haemolytic anaemia
    d. Iron deficiency anaemia (mild splenomegaly)
    e. Infantile Pyknocytosis
    f. Idiopathic myelofibrosis

3) Storage / Metabolic Disorders
    - Lipid Storage Diseases
    - Glycogen Storage Diseases
    - Mucopolysaccharidosis
    - Cholesterol Easter Storage disease
    - Amyloidosis
    - Tangier disease
    - Sea Blue Histiocyte disease
    - Galactosaemia
    - Wilson disease
    - Cystinosis
    - Fructose intolerance
    - Alpha-1 antitrypsin deficiency
    - Tyrosinaemia
    - Haemochromatosis
    - Sarchoidosis

4) Vascular Disorders
    a. Portal hypertension
        - Cirrhosis of the liver
        - Hepatitis
        - Biliary atresia
        - Cystic Fibrosis
        - Splenic Rein Thrombosis
        - Splenic Artery aneurism
        - Portal Vein Stenosis or atresia
    b. Chronic Congestive heart failure
    c. Constrictive Pericarditis

5) Tumours / Infilteration
    - Leukaemia
    - Lymphoma
    - Metastitic disease
    - Histiocytosis X
    - Splenic Haemangioma
    - Splenic cyst

6) Congenital Disorders
    - Wolman disease
    - Cockayne Syndrome
    - Miller-Dieker Syndrome
    - Dyskeratosis Congenita
    - Lysinuric Protein Intolerance
    - Beckwith Syndrome
    - Congenital Erythropoietic porphyria
    - Chediak – Higashi Syndrome
    - Familial Lipochrome Histiocytosis

7) Miscellaneous
    - Juvenile Rheumatoid Arthritis
    - SLE
    - Serum Sickness
    - Pseudosplenomegaly (downward displacement of the spleen by diaphragm)
    - Hyperparathyroidism

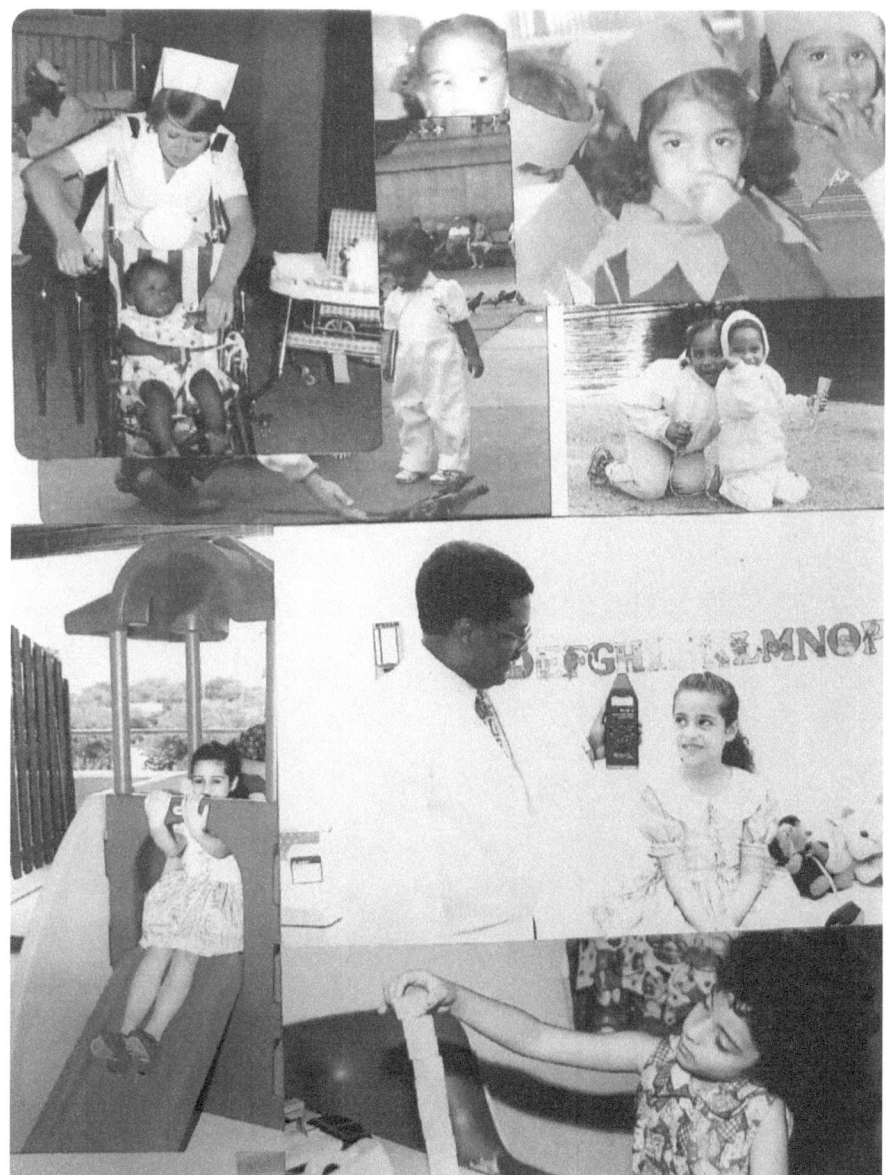

www.ingramcontent.com/pod-product-compliance
Lightning Source LLC
Chambersburg PA
CBHW020426220526
45464CB00002B/588